# THE YOGA OF INTEGRAL KNOWLEDGE

THE SYNTHESIS OF YOGA

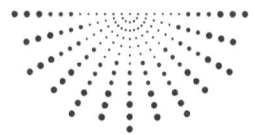

SRI AUROBINDO

# CONTENTS

## INTRODUCTION

| | |
|---|---|
| Life and Yoga | 3 |
| The Three Steps of Nature | 7 |
| The Threefold Life | 17 |
| The Systems of Yoga | 27 |
| The Synthesis of the Systems | 36 |

## THE YOGA OF INTEGRAL KNOWLEDGE

| | |
|---|---|
| The Object of Knowledge | 47 |
| The Status of Knowledge | 59 |
| The Purified Understanding | 66 |
| Concentration | 74 |
| Renunciation | 82 |
| The Synthesis of the Disciplines of Knowledge | 90 |
| The Release from Subjection to the Body | 97 |
| The Release from the Heart and the Mind | 103 |
| The Release from the Ego | 109 |
| The Realisation of the Cosmic Self | 119 |
| The Modes of the Self | 125 |
| The Realisation of Sachchidananda | 133 |
| The Difficulties of the Mental Being | 140 |
| The Passive and the Active Brahman | 148 |
| The Cosmic Consciousness | 156 |
| Oneness | 165 |
| The Soul and Nature | 171 |
| The Soul and Its Liberation | 180 |
| The Planes of Our Existence | 189 |
| The Lower Triple Purusha | 199 |
| The Ladder of Self-Transcendence | 206 |
| Vijnana or Gnosis | 215 |
| The Conditions of Attainment to the Gnosis | 226 |
| Gnosis and Ananda | 234 |
| The Higher and the Lower Knowledge | 245 |

| | |
|---|---|
| Samadhi | 252 |
| Hathayoga | 260 |
| Rajayoga | 267 |
| *Also by* SRI AUROBINDO | 275 |

# INTRODUCTION

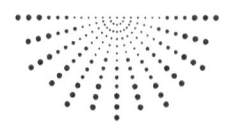

# LIFE AND YOGA

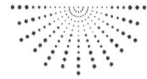

THERE are two necessities of Nature's workings which seem always to intervene in the greater forms of human activity, whether these belong to our ordinary fields of movement or seek those exceptional spheres and fulfilments which appear to us high and divine. Every such form tends towards a harmonised complexity and totality which again breaks apart into various channels of special effort and tendency, only to unite once more in a larger and more puissant synthesis. Secondly, development into forms is an imperative rule of effective manifestation; yet all truth and practice too strictly formulated becomes old and loses much, if not all, of its virtue; it must be constantly renovated by fresh streams of the spirit revivifying the dead or dying vehicle and changing it, if it is to acquire a new life. To be perpetually reborn is the condition of a material immortality. We are in an age, full of the throes of travail, when all forms of thought and activity that have in themselves any strong power of utility or any secret virtue of persistence are being subjected to a supreme test and given their opportunity of rebirth. The world today presents the aspect of a huge cauldron of Medea in which all things are being cast, shredded into pieces, experimented on, combined and recombined either to perish and provide the scattered material of new forms or to emerge rejuvenated and changed for a fresh term of existence. Indian Yoga, in its essence a special action or formulation of certain great powers of Nature, itself specialised, divided and variously formulated, is potentially one of these dynamic elements of the future life of humanity. The child of immemorial ages, preserved by its vitality and truth into our modern times, it is now emerging from the secret schools and ascetic retreats in which it had taken refuge and is seeking its place in the future sum of living human powers and utilities. But it has first to rediscover itself, bring to the surface the profoundest reason of its being in that general truth and that unceasing aim of Nature which it represents, and find by virtue of this new self-knowledge and self-appreciation its own recovered and larger synthesis. Reorganising itself, it will enter more easily and powerfully into the reorganised life of the race which its processes claim to lead within into the most secret penetralia and upward to the highest altitudes of existence and personality.

In the right view both of life and of Yoga all life is either consciously or subconsciously a Yoga. For we mean by this term a methodised effort towards self-perfection by the expression of the secret potentialities latent in the being and—highest condition of victory in that effort—a union of the human individual with the universal and transcendent Existence we see partially expressed in man and in the Cosmos. But all life, when we look behind its appearances, is a vast Yoga of Nature who attempts in the conscious and the subconscious to realise her perfection in an ever-increasing expression of her yet unrealised potentialities and to unite herself with her own divine reality. In man, her thinker, she for the first time upon this Earth devises self-conscious means and willed arrangements of activity by which this great purpose may be more swiftly and puissantly attained. Yoga, as Swami Vivekananda has said, may be regarded as a means of compressing one's evolution into a single life or a few years or even a few months of bodily existence. A given system of Yoga, then, can be no more than a selection or a compression, into narrower but more energetic forms of intensity, of the general methods which are already being used loosely, largely, in a leisurely movement, with a profuser apparent waste of material and energy but with a more complete combination by the great Mother in her vast upward labour. It is this view of Yoga that can alone form the basis for a sound and rational synthesis of Yogic methods. For then Yoga ceases to appear something mystic and abnormal which has no relation to the ordinary processes of the World-Energy or the purpose she keeps in view in her two great movements of subjective and objective self-fulfilment; it reveals itself rather as an intense and exceptional use of powers that she has already manifested or is progressively organising in her less exalted but more general operations. Yogic methods have something of the same relation to the customary psychological workings of man as has the scientific handling of the force of electricity or of steam to their normal operations in Nature. And they, too, like the operations of Science, are formed upon a knowledge developed and confirmed by regular experiment, practical analysis and constant result. All Rajayoga, for instance, depends on this perception and experience that our inner elements, combinations, functions, forces, can be separated or dissolved, can be new-combined and set to novel and formerly impossible workings or can be transformed and resolved into a new general synthesis by fixed internal processes. Hathayoga similarly depends on this perception and experience that the vital forces and functions to which our life is normally subjected and whose ordinary operations seem set and indispensable, can be mastered and the operations changed or suspended with results that would otherwise be impossible and that seem miraculous to those who have not seized the rationale of their process. And if in some other of its forms this character of Yoga is less apparent, because they are more intuitive and less mechanical, nearer, like the Yoga of Devotion, to a supernal ecstasy or, like the Yoga of Knowledge, to a supernal infinity of consciousness and being, yet they too start from the use of some principal faculty in us by ways and for ends not contemplated in its everyday spontaneous workings. All methods grouped under the common name of Yoga are special psychological processes founded on a fixed truth of Nature and developing, out of normal functions, powers and results which were always latent but which her ordinary movements do not easily or do not often manifest.

But as in physical knowledge the multiplication of scientific processes has its disadvantages, as that tends, for instance, to develop a victorious artificiality which overwhelms our natural human life under a load of machinery and to purchase certain forms of freedom and mastery at the price of an increased servitude, so the preoccupation with Yogic processes and their exceptional results may have its disadvantages and losses. The Yogin tends to draw away from the common existence and lose his hold upon it; he tends to purchase wealth of spirit by an impoverishment of his human activities, the inner freedom by an outer death. If he gains God, he loses life, or if he turns his efforts outward to conquer life, he is in danger of losing God. Therefore we see in India that a sharp incompatibility has been created between life in the world and spiritual growth and perfection, and although the tradition and ideal of a victorious harmony between the inner attraction and the outer demand remains, it is little or else very imperfectly exemplified. In fact, when a man turns his vision and energy inward and enters on the path of Yoga, he is popularly supposed to be lost inevitably to the great stream of our collective existence and the secular effort of humanity. So strongly has the idea prevailed, so much has it been emphasised by prevalent philosophies and religions that to escape from life is now commonly considered as not only the necessary condition, but the general object of Yoga. No synthesis of Yoga can be satisfying which does not, in its aim, reunite God and Nature in a liberated and perfected human life or, in its method, not only permit but favour the harmony of our inner and outer activities and experiences in the divine consummation of both. For man is precisely that term and symbol of a higher Existence descended into the material world in which it is possible for the lower to transfigure itself and put on the nature of the higher and the higher to reveal itself in the forms of the lower. To avoid the life which is given him for the realisation of that possibility, can never be either the indispensable condition or the whole and ultimate object of his supreme endeavour or of his most powerful means of self-fulfilment. It can only be a temporary necessity under certain conditions or a specialised extreme effort imposed on the individual so as to prepare a greater general possibility for the race. The true and full object and utility of Yoga can only be accomplished when the conscious Yoga in man becomes, like the subconscious Yoga in Nature, outwardly conterminous with life itself and we can once more, looking out both on the path and the achievement, say in a more perfect and luminous sense:

**"All life is Yoga."**

# THE THREE STEPS OF NATURE

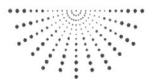

WE RECOGNISE then, in the past developments of Yoga, a specialising and separative tendency which, like all things in Nature, had its justifying and even imperative utility and we seek a synthesis of the specialised aims and methods which have, in consequence, come into being. But in order that we may be wisely guided in our effort, we must know, first, the general principle and purpose underlying this separative impulse and, next, the particular utilities upon which the method of each school of Yoga is founded. For the general principle we must interrogate the universal workings of Nature herself, recognising in her no merely specious and illusive activity of a distorting Maya, but the cosmic energy and working of God Himself in His universal being formulating and inspired by a vast, an infinite and yet a minutely selective Wisdom, *prajñā prasṛtā purāṇī* of the Upanishad, Wisdom that went forth from the Eternal since the beginning. For the particular utilities we must cast a penetrative eye on the different methods of Yoga and distinguish among the mass of their details the governing idea which they serve and the radical force which gives birth and energy to their processes of effectuation. Afterwards we may more easily find the one common principle and the one common power from which all derive their being and tendency, towards which all subconsciously move and in which, therefore, it is possible for all consciously to unite.

The progressive self-manifestation of Nature in man, termed in modern language his evolution, must necessarily depend upon three successive elements. There is that which is already evolved; there is that which, still imperfect, still partly fluid, is persistently in the stage of conscious evolution; and there is that which is to be evolved and may perhaps be already displayed, if not constantly, then occasionally or with some regularity of recurrence, in primary formations or in others more developed and, it may well be, even in some, however rare, that are near to the highest possible realisation of our present humanity. For the march of Nature is not drilled to a regular and mechanical forward stepping. She reaches constantly beyond herself even at the cost of subsequent deplorable retreats. She has rushes; she has splendid and mighty outbursts; she has immense realisations. She storms sometimes passionately forward hoping to take the kingdom of heaven by violence. And these self-exceedings are the revelation of that in her which is most divine or else most diabolical, but in either case the most puissant to bring her rapidly forward towards her goal.

That which Nature has evolved for us and has firmly founded is the bodily life. She has effected a certain combination and harmony of the two inferior but most fundamentally necessary elements of our action and progress upon earth,—Matter, which, however the too ethereally spiritual may despise it, is our foundation and the first condition of all our energies and realisations, and the Life-Energy which is our means of existence in a material body and the basis there even of our mental and spiritual activities. She has successfully achieved a certain stability of her constant material movement which is at once sufficiently steady and durable and sufficiently pliable and mutable to provide a fit dwelling-place and instrument for the progressively manifesting god in humanity. This is what is meant by the fable in the Aitareya Upanishad which tells us that the gods rejected the animal forms successively offered to them by the Divine Self and only when man was produced, cried out, "This indeed is perfectly made," and consented to enter in. She has effected also a working compromise between the inertia of matter and the active Life that lives in and feeds on it, by which not only is vital existence sustained, but the fullest developments of mentality are rendered possible. This equilibrium constitutes the basic status of Nature in man and is termed in the language of Yoga his gross body composed of the material or food sheath and the nervous system or vital vehicle.[1]

If, then, this inferior equilibrium is the basis and first means of the higher movements which the universal Power contemplates and if it constitutes the vehicle in which the Divine here seeks to reveal Itself, if the Indian saying is true that the body is the instrument provided for the fulfilment of the right law of our nature, then any final recoil from the physical life must be a turning away from the completeness of the divine Wisdom and a renunciation of its aim in earthly manifestation. Such a refusal may be, owing to some secret law of their development, the right attitude for certain individuals, but never the aim intended for mankind. It can be, therefore, no integral Yoga which ignores the body or makes its annulment or its rejection indispensable to a perfect spirituality. Rather, the perfecting of the body also should be the last triumph of the Spirit and to make the bodily life also divine must be God's final seal upon His work in the universe. The obstacle which the physical presents to the spiritual is no argument for the rejection of the physical; for in the unseen providence of things our greatest difficulties are our best opportunities. A supreme difficulty is Nature's indication to us of a supreme conquest to be won and an ultimate problem to be solved; it is not a warning of an inextricable snare to be shunned or of an enemy too strong for us from whom we must flee.

Equally, the vital and nervous energies in us are there for a great utility; they too demand the divine realisation of their possibilities in our ultimate fulfilment. The great part assigned to this element in the universal scheme is powerfully emphasised by the catholic wisdom of the Upanishads. "As the spokes of a wheel in its nave, so in the Life-Energy is all established, the triple knowledge and the Sacrifice and the power of the strong and the purity of the wise. Under the control of the LifeEnergy is all this that is established in the triple heaven."[2] It is therefore no integral Yoga that kills these vital energies, forces them into a nerveless quiescence or roots them out as the source of noxious activities. Their purification, not their destruction,—their transformation, control and utilisation is the aim in view with which they have been created and developed in us.

If the bodily life is what Nature has firmly evolved for us as her base and first instrument, it is our mental life that she is evolving as her immediate next aim and superior instrument. This in her ordinary exaltations is the lofty preoccupying thought in her; this, except in her periods of exhaustion and recoil into a reposeful and recuperating obscurity, is her constant pursuit wherever she can get free from the trammels of her first vital and physical realisations. For here in man we have a distinction which is of the utmost importance. He has in him not a single mentality, but a double and a triple, the mind material and nervous, the pure intellectual mind which liberates itself from the illusions of the body and the senses, and a divine mind above intellect which in its turn liberates itself from the imperfect modes of the logically discriminative and imaginative reason. Mind in man is first emmeshed in the life of the body, where in the plant it is entirely involved and in animals always imprisoned. It accepts this life as not only the first but the whole condition of its activities and serves its needs as if they were the entire aim of existence. But the bodily life in man is a base, not the aim, his first condition and not his last determinant. In the just idea of the ancients man is essentially the thinker, the Manu, the mental being who leads the life and the body,[3] not the animal who is led by them. The true human existence, therefore, only begins when the intellectual mentality emerges out of the material and we begin more and more to live in the mind independent of the nervous and physical obsession and in the measure of that liberty are able to accept rightly and rightly to use the life of the body. For freedom and not a skilful subjection is the true means of mastery. A free, not a compulsory acceptance of the conditions, the enlarged and sublimated conditions of our physical being, is the high human ideal. But beyond this intellectual mentality is the divine.

The mental life thus evolving in man is not, indeed, a common possession. In actual appearance it would seem as if it were only developed to the fullest in individuals and as if there were great numbers and even the majority in whom it is either a small and ill-organised part of their normal nature or not evolved at all or latent and not easily made active. Certainly, the mental life is not a finished evolution of Nature; it is not yet firmly founded in the human animal. The sign is that the fine and full equilibrium of vitality and matter, the sane, robust, long-lived human body is ordinarily found only in races or classes of men who reject the effort of thought, its disturbances, its tensions, or think only with the material mind. Civilised man has yet to establish an equilibrium between the fully active mind and the body; he does not normally possess it. Indeed, the increasing effort towards a more intense mental life seems to create, frequently, an increasing disequilibrium of the human elements, so that it is possible for eminent scientists to describe genius as a form of insanity, a result of degeneration, a pathological morbidity of Nature. The phenomena which are used to justify this exaggeration, when taken not separately, but in connection with all other relevant data, point to a different truth. Genius is one attempt of the universal Energy to so quicken and intensify our intellectual powers that they shall be prepared for those more puissant, direct and rapid faculties which constitute the play of the supra-intellectual or divine mind. It is not, then, a freak, an inexplicable phenomenon, but a perfectly natural next step in the right line of her evolution. She has harmonised the bodily life with the material mind, she is harmonising it with the play of the intellectual mentality; for that, although it tends to a depression of the full animal and vital vigour, need not produce active disturbances. And she is shooting yet beyond in the attempt to reach a still higher level. Nor are the disturbances created by her process as great as is often represented. Some of them are the crude beginnings of new manifestations; others are an easily corrected movement of disintegration, often fruitful of fresh activities and always a small price to pay for the far-reaching results that she has in view.

We may perhaps, if we consider all the circumstances, come to this conclusion that mental life, far from being a recent appearance in man, is the swift repetition in him of a previous achievement from which the Energy in the race had undergone one of her deplorable recoils. The savage is perhaps not so much the first forefather of civilised man as the degenerate descendant of a previous civilisation. For if the actuality of intellectual achievement is unevenly distributed, the capacity is spread everywhere. It has been seen that in individual cases even the racial type considered by us the lowest, the negro fresh from the perennial barbarism of Central Africa, is capable, without admixture of blood, without waiting for future generations, of the intellectual culture, if not yet of the intellectual accomplishment of the dominant European. Even in the mass men seem to need, in favourable circumstances, only a few generations to cover ground that ought apparently to be measured in the terms of millenniums. Either, then, man by his privilege as a mental being is exempt from the full burden of the tardy laws of evolution or else he already represents and with helpful conditions and in the right stimulating atmosphere can always display a high level of material capacity for the activities of the intellectual life. It is not mental incapacity, but the long rejection or seclusion from opportunity and withdrawal of the awakening impulse that creates the savage. Barbarism is an intermediate sleep, not an original darkness.

Moreover the whole trend of modern thought and modern endeavour reveals itself to the observant eye as a large conscious effort of Nature in man to effect a general level of intellectual equipment, capacity and farther possibility by universalising the opportunities which modern civilisation affords for the mental life. Even the preoccupation of the European intellect, the protagonist of this tendency, with material Nature and the externalities of existence is a necessary part of the effort. It seeks to prepare a sufficient basis in man's physical being and vital energies and in his material environment for his full mental possibilities. By the spread of education, by the advance of the backward races, by the elevation of depressed classes, by the multiplication of labour-saving appliances, by the movement towards ideal social and economic conditions, by the labour of Science towards an improved health, longevity and sound physique in civilised humanity, the sense and drift of this vast movement translates itself in easily intelligible signs. The right or at least the ultimate means may not always be employed, but their aim is the right preliminary aim,—a sound individual and social body and the satisfaction of the legitimate needs and demands of the material mind, sufficient ease, leisure, equal opportunity, so that the whole of mankind and no longer only the favoured race, class or individual may be free to develop the emotional and intellectual being to its full capacity. At present the material and economic aim may predominate, but always, behind, there works or there waits in reserve the higher and major impulse.

And when the preliminary conditions are satisfied, when the great endeavour has found its base, what will be the nature of that farther possibility which the activities of the intellectual life must serve? If Mind is indeed Nature's highest term, then the entire development of the rational and imaginative intellect and the harmonious satisfaction of the emotions and sensibilities must be to themselves sufficient. But if, on the contrary, man is more than a reasoning and emotional animal, if beyond that which is being evolved, there is something that has to be evolved, then it may well be that the fullness of the mental life, the suppleness, flexibility and wide capacity of the intellect, the ordered richness of emotion and sensibility may be only a passage towards the development of a higher life and of more powerful faculties which are yet to manifest and to take possession of the lower instrument, just as mind itself has so taken possession of the body that the physical being no longer lives only for its own satisfaction but provides the foundation and the materials for a superior activity.

The assertion of a higher than the mental life is the whole foundation of Indian philosophy and its acquisition and organisation is the veritable object served by the methods of Yoga. Mind is not the last term of evolution, not an ultimate aim, but, like body, an instrument. It is even so termed in the language of Yoga, the inner instrument.[4] And Indian tradition asserts that this which is to be manifested is not a new term in human experience, but has been developed before and has even governed humanity in certain periods of its development. In any case, in order to be known it must at one time have been partly developed. And if since then Nature has sunk back from her achievement, the reason must always be found in some unrealised harmony, some insufficiency of the intellectual and material basis to which she has now returned, some over-specialisation of the higher to the detriment of the lower existence.

But what then constitutes this higher or highest existence to which our evolution is tending? In order to answer the question we have to deal with a class of supreme experiences, a class of unusual conceptions which it is difficult to represent accurately in any other language than the ancient Sanskrit tongue in which alone they have been to some extent systematised. The only approximate terms in the English language have other associations and their use may lead to many and even serious inaccuracies. The terminology of Yoga recognises besides the status of our physical and vital being, termed the gross body and doubly composed of the food sheath and the vital vehicle, besides the status of our mental being, termed the subtle body and singly composed of the mind sheath or mental vehicle,[5] a third, supreme and divine status of supra-mental being, termed the causal body and composed of a fourth and a fifth vehicle[6] which are described as those of knowledge and bliss. But this knowledge is not a systematised result of mental questionings and reasonings, not a temporary arrangement of conclusions and opinions in the terms of the highest probability, but rather a pure self-existent and self-luminous Truth. And this bliss is not a supreme pleasure of the heart and sensations with the experience of pain and sorrow as its background, but a delight also self-existent and independent of objects and particular experiences, a self-delight which is the very nature, the very stuff, as it were, of a transcendent and infinite existence.

Do such psychological conceptions correspond to anything real and possible? All Yoga asserts them as its ultimate experience and supreme aim. They form the governing principles of our highest possible state of consciousness, our widest possible range of existence. There is, we say, a harmony of supreme faculties, corresponding roughly to the psychological faculties of revelation, inspiration and intuition, yet acting not in the intuitive reason or the divine mind, but on a still higher plane, which see Truth directly face to face, or rather live in the truth of things both universal and transcendent and are its formulation and luminous activity. And these faculties are the light of a conscious existence superseding the egoistic and itself both cosmic and transcendent, the nature of which is Bliss. These are obviously divine and, as man is at present apparently constituted, superhuman states of consciousness and activity. A trinity of transcendent existence, self-awareness and self-delight[7] is, indeed, the metaphysical description of the supreme Atman, the self-formulation, to our awakened knowledge, of the Unknowable whether conceived as a pure Impersonality or as a cosmic Personality manifesting the universe. But in Yoga they are regarded also in their psychological aspects as states of subjective existence to which our waking consciousness is now alien, but which dwell in us in a superconscious plane and to which, therefore, we may always ascend.

For, as is indicated by the name, causal body (*kāraṇa*), as opposed to the two others which are instruments (*karaṇa*), this crowning manifestation is also the source and effective power of all that in the actual evolution has preceded it. Our mental activities are, indeed, a derivation, selection and, so long as they are divided from the truth that is secretly their source, a deformation of the divine knowledge. Our sensations and emotions have the same relation to the Bliss, our vital forces and actions to the aspect of Will or Force assumed by the divine consciousness, our physical being to the pure essence of that Bliss and Consciousness. The evolution which we observe and of which we are the terrestrial summit may be considered, in a sense, as an inverse manifestation, by which these supreme Powers in their unity and their diversity use, develop and perfect the imperfect substance and activities of Matter, of Life and of Mind so that they, the inferior modes, may express in mutable relativity an increasing harmony of the divine and eternal states from which they are born. If this be the truth of the universe, then the goal of evolution is also its cause, it is that which is immanent in its elements and out of them is liberated. But the liberation is surely imperfect if it is only an escape and there is no return upon the containing substance and activities to exalt and transform them. The immanence itself would have no credible reason for being if it did not end in such a transfiguration. But if human mind can become capable of the glories of the divine Light, human emotion and sensibility can be transformed into the mould and assume the measure and movement of the supreme Bliss, human action not only represent but feel itself to be the motion of a divine and non-egoistic Force and the physical substance of our being sufficiently partake of the purity of the supernal essence, sufficiently unify plasticity and durable constancy to support and prolong these highest experiences and agencies, then all the long labour of Nature will end in a crowning justification and her evolutions reveal their profound significance.

So dazzling is even a glimpse of this supreme existence and so absorbing its attraction that, once seen, we feel readily justified in neglecting all else for its pursuit. Even, by an opposite exaggeration to that which sees all things in Mind and the mental life as an exclusive ideal, Mind comes to be regarded as an unworthy deformation and a supreme obstacle, the source of an illusory universe, a negation of the Truth and itself to be denied and all its works and results annulled if we desire the final liberation. But this is a half-truth which errs by regarding only the actual limitations of Mind and ignores its divine intention. The ultimate knowledge is that which perceives and accepts God in the universe as well as beyond the universe; the integral Yoga is that which, having found the Transcendent, can return upon the universe and possess it, retaining the power freely to descend as well as ascend the great stair of existence. For if the eternal Wisdom exists at all, the faculty of Mind also must have some high use and destiny. That use must depend on its place in the ascent and in the return and that destiny must be a fulfilment and transfiguration, not a rooting out or an annulling.

We perceive, then, these three steps in Nature, a bodily life which is the basis of our existence here in the material world, a mental life into which we emerge and by which we raise the bodily to higher uses and enlarge it into a greater completeness, and a divine existence which is at once the goal of the other two and returns upon them to liberate them into their highest possibilities. Regarding none of them as either beyond our reach or below our nature and the destruction of none of them as essential to the ultimate attainment, we accept this liberation and fulfilment as part at least and a large and important part of the aim of Yoga.

---

1. *annakoṣa* and *prāṇakoṣa*.
2. Prasna Upanishad II.
3. *manomayaḥ prāṇaśarīranetā*. Mundaka Upanishad II. 2. 8.
4. *antaḥkaraṇa*.
5. *manaḥ-koṣa*.
6. *vijñānakoṣa* and *ānandakoṣa*.
7. *saccidānanda*.

# THE THREEFOLD LIFE

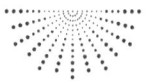

NATURE, then, is an evolution or progressive self-manifestation of an eternal and secret existence, with three successive forms as her three steps of ascent. And we have consequently as the condition of all our activities these three mutually interdependent possibilities, the bodily life, the mental existence and the veiled spiritual being which is in the involution the cause of the others and in the evolution their result. Preserving and perfecting the physical, fulfilling the mental, it is Nature's aim and it should be ours to unveil in the perfected body and mind the transcendent activities of the Spirit. As the mental life does not abrogate but works for the elevation and better utilisation of the bodily existence, so too the spiritual should not abrogate but transfigure our intellectual, emotional, aesthetic and vital activities.

For man, the head of terrestrial Nature, the sole earthly frame in which her full evolution is possible, is a triple birth. He has been given a living frame in which the body is the vessel and life the dynamic means of a divine manifestation. His activity is centred in a progressive mind which aims at perfecting itself as well as the house in which it dwells and the means of life that it uses, and is capable of awaking by a progressive self-realisation to its own true nature as a form of the Spirit. He culminates in what he always really was, the illumined and beatific spirit which is intended at last to irradiate life and mind with its now concealed splendours.

Since this is the plan of the divine Energy in humanity, the whole method and aim of our existence must work by the interaction of these three elements in the being. As a result of their separate formulation in Nature, man has open to him a choice between three kinds of life, the ordinary material existence, a life of mental activity and progress and the unchanging spiritual beatitude. But he can, as he progresses, combine these three forms, resolve their discords into a harmonious rhythm and so create in himself the whole godhead, the perfect Man.

In ordinary Nature they have each their own characteristic and governing impulse.

The characteristic energy of bodily Life is not so much in progress as in persistence, not so much in individual self-enlargement as in self-repetition. There is, indeed, in physical Nature a progression from type to type, from the vegetable to the animal, from the animal to man; for even in inanimate Matter Mind is at work. But once a type is marked off physically, the chief immediate preoccupation of the terrestrial Mother seems to be to keep it in being by a constant reproduction. For Life always seeks immortality; but since individual form is impermanent and only the idea of a form is permanent in the consciousness that creates the universe,—for there it does not perish,—such constant reproduction is the only possible material immortality. Self-preservation, self-repetition, self-multiplication are necessarily, then, the predominant instincts of all material existence. Material life seems ever to move in a fixed cycle.

The characteristic energy of pure Mind is change, and the more our mentality acquires elevation and organisation, the more this law of Mind assumes the aspect of a continual enlargement, improvement and better arrangement of its gains and so of a continual passage from a smaller and simpler to a larger and more complex perfection. For Mind, unlike bodily life, is infinite in its field, elastic in its expansion, easily variable in its formations. Change, then, self-enlargement and self-improvement are its proper instincts. Mind too moves in cycles, but these are ever-enlarging spirals. Its faith is perfectibility, its watchword is progress.

The characteristic law of Spirit is self-existent perfection and immutable infinity. It possesses always and in its own right the immortality which is the aim of Life and the perfection which is the goal of Mind. The attainment of the eternal and the realisation of that which is the same in all things and beyond all things, equally blissful in universe and outside it, untouched by the imperfections and limitations of the forms and activities in which it dwells, are the glory of the spiritual life.

In each of these forms Nature acts both individually and collectively; for the Eternal affirms Himself equally in the single form and in the group-existence, whether family, clan and nation or groupings dependent on less physical principles or the supreme group of all, our collective humanity. Man also may seek his own individual good from any or all of these spheres of activity, or identify himself in them with the collectivity and live for it, or, rising to a truer perception of this complex universe, harmonise the individual realisation with the collective aim. For as it is the right relation of the soul with the Supreme, while it is in the universe, neither to assert egoistically its separate being nor to blot itself out in the Indefinable, but to realise its unity with the Divine and the world and unite them in the individual, so the right relation of the individual with the collectivity is neither to pursue egoistically his own material or mental progress or spiritual salvation without regard to his fellows, nor for the sake of the community to suppress or maim his proper development, but to sum up in himself all its best and completest possibilities and pour them out by thought, action and all other means on his surroundings so that the whole race may approach nearer to the attainment of its supreme personalities.

It follows that the object of the material life must be to fulfil, above all things, the vital aim of Nature. The whole aim of the material man is to live, to pass from birth to death with as much comfort or enjoyment as may be on the way, but anyhow to live. He can subordinate this aim, but only to physical Nature's other instincts, the reproduction of the individual and the conservation of the type in the family, class or community. Self, domesticity, the accustomed order of the society and of the nation are the constituents of the material existence. Its immense importance in the economy of Nature is self-evident, and commensurate is the importance of the human type which represents it. He assures her of the safety of the framework she has made and of the orderly continuance and conservation of her past gains.

But by that very utility such men and the life they lead are condemned to be limited, irrationally conservative and earthbound. The customary routine, the customary institutions, the inherited or habitual forms of thought,—these things are the life-breath of their nostrils. They admit and jealously defend the changes compelled by the progressive mind in the past, but combat with equal zeal the changes that are being made by it in the present. For to the material man the living progressive thinker is an ideologue, dreamer or madman. The old Semites who stoned the living prophets and adored their memories when dead, were the very incarnation of this instinctive and unintelligent principle in Nature. In the ancient Indian distinction between the once born and the twice born, it is to this material man that the former description can be applied. He does Nature's inferior works; he assures the basis for her higher activities; but not to him easily are opened the glories of her second birth.

Yet he admits so much of spirituality as has been enforced on his customary ideas by the great religious outbursts of the past and he makes in his scheme of society a place, venerable though not often effective, for the priest or the learned theologian who can be trusted to provide him with a safe and ordinary spiritual pabulum. But to the man who would assert for himself the liberty of spiritual experience and the spiritual life, he assigns, if he admits him at all, not the vestment of the priest but the robe of the Sannyasin. Outside society let him exercise his dangerous freedom. So he may even serve as a human lightning-rod receiving the electricity of the Spirit and turning it away from the social edifice.

Nevertheless it is possible to make the material man and his life moderately progressive by imprinting on the material mind the custom of progress, the habit of conscious change, the fixed idea of progression as a law of life. The creation by this means of progressive societies in Europe is one of the greatest triumphs of Mind over Matter. But the physical nature has its revenge; for the progress made tends to be of the grosser and more outward kind and its attempts at a higher or a more rapid movement bring about great wearinesses, swift exhaustions, startling recoils.

It is possible also to give the material man and his life a moderate spirituality by accustoming him to regard in a religious spirit all the institutions of life and its customary activities. The creation of such spiritualised communities in the East has been one of the greatest triumphs of Spirit over Matter. Yet here, too, there is a defect; for this often tends only to the creation of a religious temperament, the most outward form of spirituality. Its higher manifestations, even the most splendid and puissant, either merely increase the number of souls drawn out of social life and so impoverish it or disturb the society for a while by a momentary elevation. The truth is that neither the mental effort nor the spiritual impulse can suffice, divorced from each other, to overcome the immense resistance of material Nature. She demands their alliance in a complete effort before she will suffer a complete change in humanity. But, usually, these two great agents are unwilling to make to each other the necessary concessions.

The mental life concentrates on the aesthetic, the ethical and the intellectual activities. Essential mentality is idealistic and a seeker after perfection. The subtle self, the brilliant Atman,[1] is ever a dreamer. A dream of perfect beauty, perfect conduct, perfect Truth, whether seeking new forms of the Eternal or revitalising the old, is the very soul of pure mentality. But it knows not how to deal with the resistance of Matter. There it is hampered and inefficient, works by bungling experiments and has either to withdraw from the struggle or submit to the grey actuality. Or else, by studying the material life and accepting the conditions of the contest, it may succeed, but only in imposing temporarily some artificial system which infinite Nature either rends and casts aside or disfigures out of recognition or by withdrawing her assent leaves as the corpse of a dead ideal. Few and far between have been those realisations of the dreamer in Man which the world has gladly accepted, looks back to with a fond memory and seeks, in its elements, to cherish.

When the gulf between actual life and the temperament of the thinker is too great, we see as the result a sort of withdrawing of the Mind from life in order to act with a greater freedom in its own sphere. The poet living among his brilliant visions, the artist absorbed in his art, the philosopher thinking out the problems of the intellect in his solitary chamber, the scientist, the scholar caring only for their studies and their experiments, were often in former days, are even now not unoften the Sannyasins of the intellect. To the work they have done for humanity, all its past bears record.

But such seclusion is justified only by some special activity. Mind finds fully its force and action only when it casts itself upon life and accepts equally its possibilities and its resistances as the means of a greater self-perfection. In the struggle with the difficulties of the material world the ethical development of the individual is firmly shaped and the great schools of conduct are formed; by contact with the facts of life Art attains to vitality, Thought assures its abstractions, the generalisations of the philosopher base themselves on a stable foundation of science and experience.

This mixing with life may, however, be pursued for the sake of the individual mind and with an entire indifference to the forms of the material existence or the uplifting of the race. This indifference is seen at its highest in the Epicurean discipline and is not entirely absent from the Stoic; and even altruism does the works of compassion more often for its own sake than for the sake of the world it helps. But this too is a limited fulfilment. The progressive mind is seen at its noblest when it strives to elevate the whole race to its own level whether by sowing broadcast the image of its own thought and fulfilment or by changing the material life of the race into fresh forms, religious, intellectual, social or political, intended to represent more nearly that ideal of truth, beauty, justice, righteousness with which the man's own soul is illumined. Failure in such a field matters little; for the mere attempt is dynamic and creative. The struggle of Mind to elevate life is the promise and condition of the conquest of life by that which is higher even than Mind.

That highest thing, the spiritual existence, is concerned with what is eternal but not therefore entirely aloof from the transient. For the spiritual man the mind's dream of perfect beauty is realised in an eternal love, beauty and delight that has no dependence and is equal behind all objective appearances; its dream of perfect Truth in the supreme, self-existent, self-apparent and eternal Verity which never varies, but explains and is the secret of all variations and the goal of all progress; its dream of perfect action in the omnipotent and self-guiding Law that is inherent for ever in all things and translates itself here in the rhythm of the worlds. What is fugitive vision or constant effort of creation in the brilliant Self is an eternally existing Reality in the Self that knows[2] and is the Lord.

But if it is often difficult for the mental life to accommodate itself to the dully resistant material activity, how much more difficult must it seem for the spiritual existence to live on in a world that appears full not of the Truth but of every lie and illusion, not of Love and Beauty but of an encompassing discord and ugliness, not of the Law of Truth but of victorious selfishness and sin? Therefore the spiritual life tends easily in the saint and Sannyasin to withdraw from the material existence and reject it either wholly and physically or in the spirit. It sees this world as the kingdom of evil or of ignorance and the eternal and divine either in a far-off heaven or beyond where there is no world and no life. It separates itself inwardly, if not also physically, from the world's impurities; it asserts the spiritual reality in a spotless isolation. This withdrawal renders an invaluable service to the material life itself by forcing it to regard and even to bow down to something that is the direct negation of its own petty ideals, sordid cares and egoistic self-content.

But the work in the world of so supreme a power as spiritual force cannot be thus limited. The spiritual life also can return upon the material and use it as a means of its own greater fullness. Refusing to be blinded by the dualities, the appearances, it can seek in all appearances whatsoever the vision of the same Lord, the same eternal Truth, Beauty, Love, Delight. The Vedantic formula of the Self in all things, all things in the Self and all things as becomings of the Self is the key to this richer and all-embracing Yoga.

But the spiritual life, like the mental, may thus make use of this outward existence for the benefit of the individual with a perfect indifference to any collective uplifting of the merely symbolic world which it uses. Since the Eternal is for ever the same in all things and all things the same to the Eternal, since the exact mode of action and the result are of no importance compared with the working out in oneself of the one great realisation, this spiritual indifference accepts no matter what environment, no matter what action, dispassionately, prepared to retire as soon as its own supreme end is realised. It is so that many have understood the ideal of the Gita. Or else the inner love and bliss may pour itself out on the world in good deeds, in service, in compassion, the inner Truth in the giving of knowledge, without therefore attempting the transformation of a world which must by its inalienable nature remain a battlefield of the dualities, of sin and virtue, of truth and error, of joy and suffering.

But if Progress also is one of the chief terms of world-existence and a progressive manifestation of the Divine the true sense of Nature, this limitation also is invalid. It is possible for the spiritual life in the world, and it is its real mission, to change the material life into its own image, the image of the Divine. Therefore, besides the great solitaries who have sought and attained their self-liberation, we have the great spiritual teachers who have also liberated others and, supreme of all, the great dynamic souls who, feeling themselves stronger in the might of the Spirit than all the forces of the material life banded together, have thrown themselves upon the world, grappled with it in a loving wrestle and striven to compel its consent to its own transfiguration. Ordinarily, the effort is concentrated on a mental and moral change in humanity, but it may extend itself also to the alteration of the forms of our life and its institutions so that they too may be a better mould for the inpourings of the Spirit. These attempts have been the supreme landmarks in the progressive development of human ideals and the divine preparation of the race. Every one of them, whatever its outward results, has left Earth more capable of Heaven and quickened in its tardy movements the evolutionary Yoga of Nature.

In India, for the last thousand years and more, the spiritual life and the material have existed side by side to the exclusion of the progressive mind. Spirituality has made terms for itself with Matter by renouncing the attempt at general progress. It has obtained from society the right of free spiritual development for all who assume some distinctive symbol, such as the garb of the Sannyasin, the recognition of that life as man's goal and those who live it as worthy of an absolute reverence, and the casting of society itself into such a religious mould that its most customary acts should be accompanied by a formal reminder of the spiritual symbolism of life and its ultimate destination. On the other hand, there was conceded to society the right of inertia and immobile self-conservation. The concession destroyed much of the value of the terms. The religious mould being fixed, the formal reminder tended to become a routine and to lose its living sense. The constant attempts to change the mould by new sects and religions ended only in a new routine or a modification of the old; for the saving element of the free and active mind had been exiled. The material life, handed over to the Ignorance, the purposeless and endless duality, became a leaden and dolorous yoke from which flight was the only escape.

The schools of Indian Yoga lent themselves to the compromise. Individual perfection or liberation was made the aim, seclusion of some kind from the ordinary activities the condition, the renunciation of life the culmination. The teacher gave his knowledge only to a small circle of disciples. Or if a wider movement was attempted, it was still the release of the individual soul that remained the aim. The pact with an immobile society was, for the most part, observed.

The utility of the compromise in the then actual state of the world cannot be doubted. It secured in India a society which lent itself to the preservation and the worship of spirituality, a country apart in which as in a fortress the highest spiritual ideal could maintain itself in its most absolute purity unoverpowered by the siege of the forces around it. But it was a compromise, not an absolute victory. The material life lost the divine impulse to growth, the spiritual preserved by isolation its height and purity, but sacrificed its full power and serviceableness to the world. Therefore, in the divine Providence the country of the Yogins and the Sannyasins has been forced into a strict and imperative contact with the very element it had rejected, the element of the progressive Mind, so that it might recover what was now wanting to it.

We have to recognise once more that the individual exists not in himself alone but in the collectivity and that individual perfection and liberation are not the whole sense of God's intention in the world. The free use of our liberty includes also the liberation of others and of mankind; the perfect utility of our perfection is, having realised in ourselves the divine symbol, to reproduce, multiply and ultimately universalise it in others.

Therefore from a concrete view of human life in its threefold potentialities we come to the same conclusion that we had drawn from an observation of Nature in her general workings and the three steps of her evolution. And we begin to perceive a complete aim for our synthesis of Yoga.

Spirit is the crown of universal existence; Matter is its basis; Mind is the link between the two. Spirit is that which is eternal; Mind and Matter are its workings. Spirit is that which is concealed and has to be revealed; mind and body are the means by which it seeks to reveal itself. Spirit is the image of the Lord of the Yoga; mind and body are the means He has provided for reproducing that image in phenomenal existence. All Nature is an attempt at a progressive revelation of the concealed Truth, a more and more successful reproduction of the divine image.

But what Nature aims at for the mass in a slow evolution, Yoga effects for the individual by a rapid revolution. It works by a quickening of all her energies, a sublimation of all her faculties. While she develops the spiritual life with difficulty and has constantly to fall back from it for the sake of her lower realisations, the sublimated force, the concentrated method of Yoga can attain directly and carry with it the perfection of the mind and even, if she will, the perfection of the body. Nature seeks the Divine in her own symbols: Yoga goes beyond Nature to the Lord of Nature, beyond universe to the Transcendent and can return with the transcendent light and power, with the fiat of the Omnipotent.

But their aim is one in the end. The generalisation of Yoga in humanity must be the last victory of Nature over her own delays and concealments. Even as now by the progressive mind in Science she seeks to make all mankind fit for the full development of the mental life, so by Yoga must she inevitably seek to make all mankind fit for the higher evolution, the second birth, the spiritual existence. And as the mental life uses and perfects the material, so will the spiritual use and perfect the material and the mental existence as the instruments of a divine self-expression. The ages when that is accomplished, are the legendary Satya or Krita[3] Yugas, the ages of the Truth manifested in the symbol, of the great work done when Nature in mankind, illumined, satisfied and blissful, rests in the culmination of her endeavour.

It is for man to know her meaning, no longer misunderstanding, vilifying or misusing the universal Mother, and to aspire always by her mightiest means to her highest ideal.

---

1. Who dwells in Dream, the inly conscious, the enjoyer of abstractions, the Brilliant. Mandukya Upanishad 4.
2. The Unified, in whom conscious thought is concentrated, who is all delight and enjoyer of delight, the Wise. . . . He is the Lord of all, the Omniscient, the inner Guide. Mandukya Upanishad 5, 6.
3. Satya means Truth; Krita, effected or completed.

# THE SYSTEMS OF YOGA

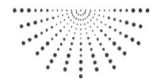

THESE relations between the different psychological divisions of the human being and these various utilities and objects of effort founded on them, such as we have seen them in our brief survey of the natural evolution, we shall find repeated in the fundamental principles and methods of the different schools of Yoga. And if we seek to combine and harmonise their central practices and their predominant aims, we shall find that the basis provided by Nature is still our natural basis and the condition of their synthesis.

In one respect Yoga exceeds the normal operation of cosmic Nature and climbs beyond her. For the aim of the Universal Mother is to embrace the Divine in her own play and creations and there to realise It. But in the highest flights of Yoga she reaches beyond herself and realises the Divine in Itself exceeding the universe and even standing apart from the cosmic play. Therefore by some it is supposed that this is not only the highest but also the one true or exclusively preferable object of Yoga.

Yet it is always through something which she has formed in her evolution that Nature thus overpasses her evolution. It is the individual heart that by sublimating its highest and purest emotions attains to the transcendent Bliss or the ineffable Nirvana, the individual mind that by converting its ordinary functionings into a knowledge beyond mentality knows its oneness with the Ineffable and merges its separate existence in that transcendent unity. And always it is the individual, the Self conditioned in its experience by Nature and working through her formations, that attains to the Self unconditioned, free and transcendent.

In practice three conceptions are necessary before there can be any possibility of Yoga; there must be, as it were, three consenting parties to the effort,—God, Nature and the human soul or, in more abstract language, the Transcendental, the Universal and the Individual. If the individual and Nature are left to themselves, the one is bound to the other and unable to exceed appreciably her lingering march. Something transcendent is needed, free from her and greater, which will act upon us and her, attracting us upward to Itself and securing from her by good grace or by force her consent to the individual ascension.

It is this truth which makes necessary to every philosophy of Yoga the conception of the Ishwara, Lord, supreme Soul or supreme Self, towards whom the effort is directed and who gives the illuminating touch and the strength to attain. Equally true is the complementary idea so often enforced by the Yoga of devotion that as the Transcendent is necessary to the individual and sought after by him, so also the individual is necessary in a sense to the Transcendent and sought after by It. If the Bhakta seeks and yearns after Bhagavan, Bhagavan also seeks and yearns after the Bhakta.[1] There can be no Yoga of knowledge without a human seeker of the knowledge, the supreme subject of knowledge and the divine use by the individual of the universal faculties of knowledge; no Yoga of devotion without the human God-lover, the supreme object of love and delight and the divine use by the individual of the universal faculties of spiritual, emotional and aesthetic enjoyment; no Yoga of works without the human worker, the supreme Will, Master of all works and sacrifices, and the divine use by the individual of the universal faculties of power and action. However Monistic may be our intellectual conception of the highest truth of things, in practice we are compelled to accept this omnipresent Trinity.

For the contact of the human and individual consciousness with the divine is the very essence of Yoga. Yoga is the union of that which has become separated in the play of the universe with its own true self, origin and universality. The contact may take place at any point of the complex and intricately organised consciousness which we call our personality. It may be effected in the physical through the body; in the vital through the action of those functionings which determine the state and the experiences of our nervous being; through the mentality, whether by means of the emotional heart, the active will or the understanding mind, or more largely by a general conversion of the mental consciousness in all its activities. It may equally be accomplished through a direct awakening to the universal or transcendent Truth and Bliss by the conversion of the central ego in the mind. And according to the point of contact that we choose will be the type of the Yoga that we practise.

For if, leaving aside the complexities of their particular processes, we fix our regard on the central principle of the chief schools of Yoga still prevalent in India, we find that they arrange themselves in an ascending order which starts from the lowest rung of the ladder, the body, and ascends to the direct contact between the individual soul and the transcendent and universal Self. Hathayoga selects the body and the vital functionings as its instruments of perfection and realisation; its concern is with the gross body. Rajayoga selects the mental being in its different parts as its lever-power; it concentrates on the subtle body. The triple Path of Works, of Love and of Knowledge uses some part of the mental being, will, heart or intellect as a starting-point and seeks by its conversion to arrive at the liberating Truth, Beatitude and Infinity which are the nature of the spiritual life. Its method is a direct commerce between the human Purusha in the individual body and the divine Purusha who dwells in every body and yet transcends all form and name.

Hathayoga aims at the conquest of the life and the body whose combination in the food sheath and the vital vehicle constitutes, as we have seen, the gross body and whose equilibrium is the foundation of all Nature's workings in the human being. The equilibrium established by Nature is sufficient for the normal egoistic life; it is insufficient for the purpose of the Hathayogin. For it is calculated on the amount of vital or dynamic force necessary to drive the physical engine during the normal span of human life and to perform more or less adequately the various workings demanded of it by the individual life inhabiting this frame and the world-environment by which it is conditioned.

Hathayoga therefore seeks to rectify Nature and establish another equilibrium by which the physical frame will be able to sustain the inrush of an increasing vital or dynamic force of Prana indefinite, almost infinite in its quantity or intensity. In Nature the equilibrium is based upon the individualisation of a limited quantity and force of the Prana; more than that the individual is by personal and hereditary habit unable to bear, use or control. In Hathayoga, the equilibrium opens a door to the universalisation of the individual vitality by admitting into the body, containing, using and controlling a much less fixed and limited action of the universal energy.

The chief processes of Hathayoga are *āsana* and *prāṇāyāma*. By its numerous *āsanas* or fixed postures it first cures the body of that restlessness which is a sign of its inability to contain without working them off in action and movement the vital forces poured into it from the universal Life-Ocean, gives to it an extraordinary health, force and suppleness and seeks to liberate it from the habits by which it is subjected to ordinary physical Nature and kept within the narrow bounds of her normal operations. In the ancient tradition of Hathayoga it has always been supposed that this conquest could be pushed so far even as to conquer to a great extent the force of gravitation. By various subsidiary but elaborate processes the Hathayogin next contrives to keep the body free from all impurities and the nervous system unclogged for those exercises of respiration which are his most important instruments. These are called *prāṇāyāma*, the control of the breath or vital power; for breathing is the chief physical functioning of the vital forces. Pranayama, for the Hathayogin, serves a double purpose. First, it completes the perfection of the body. The vitality is liberated from many of the ordinary necessities of physical Nature; robust health, prolonged youth, often an extraordinary longevity are attained. On the other hand, Pranayama awakens the coiled-up serpent of the Pranic dynamism in the vital sheath and opens to the Yogin fields of consciousness, ranges of experience, abnormal faculties denied to the ordinary human life while it puissantly intensifies such normal powers and faculties as he already possesses.

These advantages can be farther secured and emphasised by other subsidiary processes open to the Hathayogin.

The results of Hathayoga are thus striking to the eye and impose easily on the vulgar or physical mind. And yet at the end we may ask what we have gained at the end of all this stupendous labour. The object of physical Nature, the preservation of the mere physical life, its highest perfection, even in a certain sense the capacity of a greater enjoyment of physical living have been carried out on an abnormal scale. But the weakness of Hathayoga is that its laborious and difficult processes make so great a demand on the time and energy and impose so complete a severance from the ordinary life of men that the utilisation of its results for the life of the world becomes either impracticable or is extraordinarily restricted. If in return for this loss we gain another life in another world within, the mental, the dynamic, these results could have been acquired through other systems, through Rajayoga, through Tantra, by much less laborious methods and held on much less exacting terms. On the other hand the physical results, increased vitality, prolonged youth, health, longevity are of small avail if they must be held by us as misers of ourselves, apart from the common life, for their own sake, not utilised, not thrown into the common sum of the world's activities. Hathayoga attains large results, but at an exorbitant price and to very little purpose.

Rajayoga takes a higher flight. It aims at the liberation and perfection not of the bodily, but of the mental being, the control of the emotional and sensational life, the mastery of the whole apparatus of thought and consciousness. It fixes its eyes on the *citta*, that stuff of mental consciousness in which all these activities arise, and it seeks, even as Hathayoga with its physical material, first to purify and to tranquillise. The normal state of man is a condition of trouble and disorder, a kingdom either at war with itself or badly governed; for the lord, the Purusha, is subjected to his ministers, the faculties, subjected even to his subjects, the instruments of sensation, emotion, action, enjoyment. Swarajya, self-rule, must be substituted for this subjection. First, therefore, the powers of order must be helped to overcome the powers of disorder. The preliminary movement of Rajayoga is a careful self-discipline by which good habits of mind are substituted for the lawless movements that indulge the lower nervous being. By the practice of truth, by renunciation of all forms of egoistic seeking, by abstention from injury to others, by purity, by constant meditation and inclination to the divine Purusha who is the true lord of the mental kingdom, a pure, glad, clear state of mind and heart is established.

This is the first step only. Afterwards, the ordinary activities of the mind and sense must be entirely quieted in order that the soul may be free to ascend to higher states of consciousness and acquire the foundation for a perfect freedom and self-mastery. But Rajayoga does not forget that the disabilities of the ordinary mind proceed largely from its subjection to the reactions of the nervous system and the body. It adopts therefore from the Hathayogic system its devices of *āsana* and *prāṇāyāma*, but reduces their multiple and elaborate forms in each case to one simplest and most directly effective process sufficient for its own immediate object. Thus it gets rid of the Hathayogic complexity and cumbrousness while it utilises the swift and powerful efficacy of its methods for the control of the body and the vital functions and for the awakening of that internal dynamism, full of a latent supernormal faculty, typified in Yogic terminology by the *kuṇḍalinī*, the coiled and sleeping serpent of Energy within. This done, the system proceeds to the perfect quieting of the restless mind and its elevation to a higher plane through concentration of mental force by the successive stages which lead to the utmost inner concentration or ingathered state of the consciousness which is called Samadhi.

By Samadhi, in which the mind acquires the capacity of withdrawing from its limited waking activities into freer and higher states of consciousness, Rajayoga serves a double purpose. It compasses a pure mental action liberated from the confusions of the outer consciousness and passes thence to the higher supra-mental planes on which the individual soul enters into its true spiritual existence. But also it acquires the capacity of that free and concentrated energising of consciousness on its object which our philosophy asserts as the primary cosmic energy and the method of divine action upon the world. By this capacity the Yogin, already possessed of the highest supracosmic knowledge and experience in the state of trance, is able in the waking state to acquire directly whatever knowledge and exercise whatever mastery may be useful or necessary to his activities in the objective world. For the ancient system of Rajayoga aimed not only at Swarajya, self-rule or subjective empire, the entire control by the subjective consciousness of all the states and activities proper to its own domain, but included Samrajya as well, outward empire, the control by the subjective consciousness of its outer activities and environment.

We perceive that as Hathayoga, dealing with the life and body, aims at the supernormal perfection of the physical life and its capacities and goes beyond it into the domain of the mental life, so Rajayoga, operating with the mind, aims at a supernormal perfection and enlargement of the capacities of the mental life and goes beyond it into the domain of the spiritual existence. But the weakness of the system lies in its excessive reliance on abnormal states of trance. This limitation leads first to a certain aloofness from the physical life which is our foundation and the sphere into which we have to bring our mental and spiritual gains. Especially is the spiritual life, in this system, too much associated with the state of Samadhi. Our object is to make the spiritual life and its experiences fully active and fully utilisable in the waking state and even in the normal use of the functions. But in Rajayoga it tends to withdraw into a subliminal plane at the back of our normal experiences instead of descending and possessing our whole existence.

The triple Path of devotion, knowledge and works attempts the province which Rajayoga leaves unoccupied. It differs from Rajayoga in that it does not occupy itself with the elaborate training of the whole mental system as the condition of perfection, but seizes on certain central principles, the intellect, the heart, the will, and seeks to convert their normal operations by turning them away from their ordinary and external preoccupation and activities and concentrating them on the Divine. It differs also in this,—and here from the point of view of an integral Yoga there seems to be a defect,—that it is indifferent to mental and bodily perfection and aims only at purity as a condition of the divine realisation. A second defect is that as actually practised it chooses one of the three parallel paths exclusively and almost in antagonism to the others instead of effecting a synthetic harmony of the intellect, the heart and the will in an integral divine realisation.

The Path of Knowledge aims at the realisation of the unique and supreme Self. It proceeds by the method of intellectual reflection, *vicāra*, to right discrimination, *viveka*. It observes and distinguishes the different elements of our apparent or phenomenal being and rejecting identification with each of them arrives at their exclusion and separation in one common term as constituents of Prakriti, of phenomenal Nature, creations of Maya, the phenomenal consciousness. So it is able to arrive at its right identification with the pure and unique Self which is not mutable or perishable, not determinable by any phenomenon or combination of phenomena. From this point the path, as ordinarily followed, leads to the rejection of the phenomenal worlds from the consciousness as an illusion and the final immergence without return of the individual soul in the Supreme.

But this exclusive consummation is not the sole or inevitable result of the Path of Knowledge. For, followed more largely and with a less individual aim, the method of Knowledge may lead to an active conquest of the cosmic existence for the Divine no less than to a transcendence. The point of this departure is the realisation of the supreme Self not only in one's own being but in all beings and, finally, the realisation of even the phenomenal aspects of the world as a play of the divine consciousness and not something entirely alien to its true nature. And on the basis of this realisation a yet further enlargement is possible, the conversion of all forms of knowledge, however mundane, into activities of the divine consciousness utilisable for the perception of the one and unique Object of knowledge both in itself and through the play of its forms and symbols. Such a method might well lead to the elevation of the whole range of human intellect and perception to the divine level, to its spiritualisation and to the justification of the cosmic travail of knowledge in humanity. The Path of Devotion aims at the enjoyment of the supreme Love and Bliss and utilises normally the conception of the supreme Lord in His personality as the divine Lover and enjoyer of the universe. The world is then realised as a play of the Lord, with our human life as its final stage, pursued through the different phases of self-concealment and self-revelation. The principle of Bhakti Yoga is to utilise all the normal relations of human life into which emotion enters and apply them no longer to transient worldly relations, but to the joy of the All-Loving, the All-Beautiful and the All-Blissful. Worship and meditation are used only for the preparation and increase of intensity of the divine relationship. And this Yoga is catholic in its use of all emotional relations, so that even enmity and opposition to God, considered as an intense, impatient and perverse form of Love, is conceived as a possible means of realisation and salvation. This path, too, as ordinarily practised, leads away from world-existence to an absorption, of another kind than the Monist's, in the Transcendent and Supra-cosmic.

But, here too, the exclusive result is not inevitable. The Yoga itself provides a first corrective by not confining the play of divine love to the relation between the supreme Soul and the individual, but extending it to a common feeling and mutual worship between the devotees themselves united in the same realisation of the supreme Love and Bliss. It provides a yet more general corrective in the realisation of the divine object of Love in all beings not only human but animal, easily extended to all forms whatsoever. We can see how this larger application of the Yoga of Devotion may be so used as to lead to the elevation of the whole range of human emotion, sensation and aesthetic perception to the divine level, its spiritualisation and the justification of the cosmic labour towards love and joy in our humanity.

The Path of Works aims at the dedication of every human activity to the supreme Will. It begins by the renunciation of all egoistic aim for our works, all pursuit of action for an interested aim or for the sake of a worldly result. By this renunciation it so purifies the mind and the will that we become easily conscious of the great universal Energy as the true doer of all our actions and the Lord of that Energy as their ruler and director with the individual as only a mask, an excuse, an instrument or, more positively, a conscious centre of action and phenomenal relation. The choice and direction of the act is more and more consciously left to this supreme Will and this universal Energy. To That our works as well as the results of our works are finally abandoned. The object is the release of the soul from its bondage to appearances and to the reaction of phenomenal activities. Karmayoga is used, like the other paths, to lead to liberation from phenomenal existence and a departure into the Supreme. But here too the exclusive result is not inevitable. The end of the path may be, equally, a perception of the Divine in all energies, in all happenings, in all activities, and a free and unegoistic participation of the soul in the cosmic action. So followed it will lead to the elevation of all human will and activity to the divine level, its spiritualisation and the justification of the cosmic labour towards freedom, power and perfection in the human being.

We can see also that in the integral view of things these three paths are one. Divine Love should normally lead to the perfect knowledge of the Beloved by perfect intimacy, thus becoming a path of Knowledge, and to divine service, thus becoming a path of Works. So also should perfect Knowledge lead to perfect Love and Joy and a full acceptance of the works of That which is known; dedicated Works to the entire love of the Master of the Sacrifice and the deepest knowledge of His ways and His being. It is in this triple path that we come most readily to the absolute knowledge, love and service of the One in all beings and in the entire cosmic manifestation.

---

1. Bhakta, the devotee or lover of God; Bhagavan, God, the Lord of Love and Delight. The third term of the trinity is Bhagavat, the divine revelation of Love.

# THE SYNTHESIS OF THE SYSTEMS

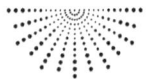

BY THE very nature of the principal Yogic schools, each covering in its operations a part of the complex human integer and attempting to bring out its highest possibilities, it will appear that a synthesis of all of them largely conceived and applied might well result in an integral Yoga. But they are so disparate in their tendencies, so highly specialised and elaborated in their forms, so long confirmed in the mutual opposition of their ideas and methods that we do not easily find how we can arrive at their right union.

An undiscriminating combination in block would not be a synthesis, but a confusion. Nor would a successive practice of each of them in turn be easy in the short span of our human life and with our limited energies, to say nothing of the waste of labour implied in so cumbrous a process. Sometimes, indeed, Hathayoga and Rajayoga are thus successively practised. And in a recent unique example, in the life of Ramakrishna Paramhansa, we see a colossal spiritual capacity first driving straight to the divine realisation, taking, as it were, the kingdom of heaven by violence, and then seizing upon one Yogic method after another and extracting the substance out of it with an incredible rapidity, always to return to the heart of the whole matter, the realisation and possession of God by the power of love, by the extension of inborn spirituality into various experience and by the spontaneous play of an intuitive knowledge. Such an example cannot be generalised. Its object also was special and temporal, to exemplify in the great and decisive experience of a master-soul the truth, now most necessary to humanity, towards which a world long divided into jarring sects and schools is with difficulty labouring, that all sects are forms and fragments of a single integral truth and all disciplines labour in their different ways towards one supreme experience. To know, be and possess the Divine is the one thing needful and it includes or leads up to all the rest; towards this sole good we have to drive and this attained, all the rest that the divine Will chooses for us, all necessary form and manifestation, will be added.

The synthesis we propose cannot, then, be arrived at either by combination in mass or by successive practice. It must therefore be effected by neglecting the forms and outsides of the Yogic disciplines and seizing rather on some central principle common to all which will include and utilise in the right place and proportion their particular principles, and on some central dynamic force which is the common secret of their divergent methods and capable therefore of organising a natural selection and combination of their varied energies and different utilities. This was the aim which we set before ourselves at first when we entered upon our comparative examination of the methods of Nature and the methods of Yoga and we now return to it with the possibility of hazarding some definite solution.

We observe, first, that there still exists in India a remarkable Yogic system which is in its nature synthetical and starts from a great central principle of Nature, a great dynamic force of Nature; but it is a Yoga apart, not a synthesis of other schools. This system is the way of the Tantra. Owing to certain of its developments Tantra has fallen into discredit with those who are not Tantrics; and especially owing to the developments of its left-hand path, the Vama Marga, which not content with exceeding the duality of virtue and sin and instead of replacing them by spontaneous rightness of action seemed, sometimes, to make a method of self-indulgence, a method of unrestrained social immorality. Nevertheless, in its origin, Tantra was a great and puissant system founded upon ideas which were at least partially true. Even its twofold division into the right-hand and left-hand paths, Dakshina Marga and Vama Marga, started from a certain profound perception. In the ancient symbolic sense of the words Dakshina and Vama, it was the distinction between the way of Knowledge and the way of Ananda,—Nature in man liberating itself by right discrimination in power and practice of its own energies, elements and potentialities and Nature in man liberating itself by joyous acceptance in power and practice of its own energies, elements and potentialities. But in both paths there was in the end an obscuration of principles, a deformation of symbols and a fall.

If, however, we leave aside, here also, the actual methods and practices and seek for the central principle, we find, first, that Tantra expressly differentiates itself from the Vedic methods of Yoga. In a sense, all the schools we have hitherto examined are Vedantic in their principle; their force is in knowledge, their method is knowledge, though it is not always discernment by the intellect, but may be, instead, the knowledge of the heart expressed in love and faith or a knowledge in the will working out through action. In all of them the lord of the Yoga is the Purusha, the Conscious Soul that knows, observes, attracts, governs. But in Tantra it is rather Prakriti, the Nature-Soul, the Energy, the Will-in-Power executive in the universe. It was by learning and applying the intimate secrets of this Will-in-Power, its method, its Tantra, that the Tantric Yogin pursued the aims of his discipline,—mastery, perfection, liberation, beatitude. Instead of drawing back from manifested Nature and its difficulties, he confronted them, seized and conquered. But in the end, as is the general tendency of Prakriti, Tantric Yoga largely lost its principle in its machinery and became a thing of formulae and occult mechanism still powerful when rightly used but fallen from the clarity of their original intention.

We have in this central Tantric conception one side of the truth, the worship of the Energy, the Shakti, as the sole effective force for all attainment. We get the other extreme in the Vedantic conception of the Shakti as a power of Illusion and in the search after the silent inactive Purusha as the means of liberation from the deceptions created by the active Energy. But in the integral conception the Conscious Soul is the Lord, the Nature-Soul is his executive Energy. Purusha is of the nature of Sat, the being of conscious self-existence pure and infinite; Shakti or Prakriti is of the nature of Chit,—it is power of the Purusha's self-conscious existence, pure and infinite. The relation of the two exists between the poles of rest and action. When the Energy is absorbed in the bliss of conscious self-existence, there is rest; when the Purusha pours itself out in the action of its Energy, there is action, creation and the enjoyment or Ananda of becoming. But if Ananda is the creator and begetter of all becoming, its method is Tapas or force of the Purusha's consciousness dwelling upon its own infinite potentiality in existence and producing from it truths of conception or real Ideas, *vijñāna*, which, proceeding from an omniscient and omnipotent Self-existence, have the surety of their own fulfilment and contain in themselves the nature and law of their own becoming in the terms of mind, life and matter. The eventual omnipotence of Tapas and the infallible fulfilment of the Idea are the very foundation of all Yoga. In man we render these terms by Will and Faith,—a will that is eventually self-effective because it is of the substance of Knowledge and a faith that is the reflex in the lower consciousness of a Truth or real Idea yet unrealised in the manifestation. It is this self-certainty of the Idea which is meant by the Gita when it says, *yo yac-chraddhaḥ sa eva saḥ* , "whatever is a man's faith or the sure Idea in him, that he becomes."

We see, then, what from the psychological point of view,—and Yoga is nothing but practical psychology,—is the conception of Nature from which we have to start. It is the self-fulfilment of the Purusha through his Energy. But the movement of Nature is twofold, higher and lower, or, as we may choose to term it, divine and undivine. The distinction exists indeed for practical purposes only; for there is nothing that is not divine, and in a larger view it is as meaningless, verbally, as the distinction between natural and supernatural, for all things that are are natural. All things are in Nature and all things are in God. But, for practical purposes, there is a real distinction. The lower Nature, that which we know and are and must remain so long as the faith in us is not changed, acts through limitation and division, is of the nature of Ignorance and culminates in the life of the ego; but the higher Nature, that to which we aspire, acts by unification and transcendence of limitation, is of the nature of Knowledge and culminates in the life divine. The passage from the lower to the higher is the aim of Yoga; and this passage may effect itself by the rejection of the lower and escape into the higher,—the ordinary view-point,—or by the transformation of the lower and its elevation to the higher Nature. It is this, rather, that must be the aim of an integral Yoga.

But in either case it is always through something in the lower that we must rise into the higher existence, and the schools of Yoga each select their own point of departure or their own gate of escape. They specialise certain activities of the lower Prakriti and turn them towards the Divine. But the normal action of Nature in us is an integral movement in which the full complexity of all our elements is affected by and affects all our environments. The whole of life is the Yoga of Nature. The Yoga that we seek must also be an integral action of Nature, and the whole difference between the Yogin and the natural man will be this, that the Yogin seeks to substitute in himself for the integral action of the lower Nature working in and by ego and division the integral action of the higher Nature working in and by God and unity. If indeed our aim be only an escape from the world to God, synthesis is unnecessary and a waste of time; for then our sole practical aim must be to find out one path out of the thousand that lead to God, one shortest possible of short cuts, and not to linger exploring different paths that end in the same goal. But if our aim be a transformation of our integral being into the terms of God-existence, it is then that a synthesis becomes necessary.

The method we have to pursue, then, is to put our whole conscious being into relation and contact with the Divine and to call Him in to transform our entire being into His. Thus in a sense God Himself, the real Person in us, becomes the sadhaka of the sadhana[1] as well as the Master of the Yoga by whom the lower personality is used as the centre of a divine transfiguration and the instrument of its own perfection. In effect, the pressure of the Tapas, the force of consciousness in us dwelling in the Idea of the divine Nature upon that which we are in our entirety, produces its own realisation. The divine and all-knowing and all-effecting descends upon the limited and obscure, progressively illumines and energises the whole lower nature and substitutes its own action for all the terms of the inferior human light and mortal activity.

In psychological fact this method translates itself into the progressive surrender of the ego with its whole field and all its apparatus to the Beyond-ego with its vast and incalculable but always inevitable workings. Certainly, this is no short cut or easy sadhana. It requires a colossal faith, an absolute courage and above all an unflinching patience. For it implies three stages of which only the last can be wholly blissful or rapid,—the attempt of the ego to enter into contact with the Divine, the wide, full and therefore laborious preparation of the whole lower Nature by the divine working to receive and become the higher Nature, and the eventual transformation. In fact, however, the divine Strength, often unobserved and behind the veil, substitutes itself for our weakness and supports us through all our failings of faith, courage and patience. It "makes the blind to see and the lame to stride over the hills." The intellect becomes aware of a Law that beneficently insists and a succour that upholds; the heart speaks of a Master of all things and Friend of man or a universal Mother who upholds through all stumblings. Therefore this path is at once the most difficult imaginable and yet, in comparison with the magnitude of its effort and object, the most easy and sure of all.

There are three outstanding features of this action of the higher when it works integrally on the lower nature. In the first place it does not act according to a fixed system and succession as in the specialised methods of Yoga, but with a sort of free, scattered and yet gradually intensive and purposeful working determined by the temperament of the individual in whom it operates, the helpful materials which his nature offers and the obstacles which it presents to purification and perfection. In a sense, therefore, each man in this path has his own method of Yoga. Yet are there certain broad lines of working common to all which enable us to construct not indeed a routine system, but yet some kind of Shastra or scientific method of the synthetic Yoga.

Secondly, the process, being integral, accepts our nature such as it stands organised by our past evolution and without rejecting anything essential compels all to undergo a divine change. Everything in us is seized by the hands of a mighty Artificer and transformed into a clear image of that which it now seeks confusedly to present. In that ever-progressive experience we begin to perceive how this lower manifestation is constituted and that everything in it, however seemingly deformed or petty or vile, is the more or less distorted or imperfect figure of some element or action in the harmony of the divine Nature. We begin to understand what the Vedic Rishis meant when they spoke of the human forefathers fashioning the gods as a smith forges the crude material in his smithy.

Thirdly, the divine Power in us uses all life as the means of this integral Yoga. Every experience and outer contact with our world-environment, however trifling or however disastrous, is used for the work, and every inner experience, even to the most repellent suffering or the most humiliating fall, becomes a step on the path to perfection. And we recognise in ourselves with opened eyes the method of God in the world, His purpose of light in the obscure, of might in the weak and fallen, of delight in what is grievous and miserable. We see the divine method to be the same in the lower and in the higher working; only in the one it is pursued tardily and obscurely through the subconscious in Nature, in the other it becomes swift and self-conscious and the instrument confesses the hand of the Master. All life is a Yoga of Nature seeking to manifest God within itself. Yoga marks the stage at which this effort becomes capable of self-awareness and therefore of right completion in the individual. It is a gathering up and concentration of the movements dispersed and loosely combined in the lower evolution.

An integral method and an integral result. First, an integral realisation of Divine Being; not only a realisation of the One in its indistinguishable unity, but also in its multitude of aspects which are also necessary to the complete knowledge of it by the relative consciousness; not only realisation of unity in the Self, but of unity in the infinite diversity of activities, worlds and creatures.

Therefore, also, an integral liberation. Not only the freedom born of unbroken contact and identification of the individual being in all its parts with the Divine, *sāyujya-mukti*, by which it can become free[2] even in its separation, even in the duality; not only the *sālokya-mukti* by which the whole conscious existence dwells in the same status of being as the Divine, in the state of Sachchidananda; but also the acquisition of the divine nature by the transformation of this lower being into the human image of the Divine, *sādharmya-mukti*, and the complete and final release of all, the liberation of the consciousness from the transitory mould of the ego and its unification with the One Being, universal both in the world and the individual and transcendentally one both in the world and beyond all universe.

By this integral realisation and liberation, the perfect harmony of the results of Knowledge, Love and Works. For there is attained the complete release from ego and identification in being with the One in all and beyond all. But since the attaining consciousness is not limited by its attainment, we win also the unity in Beatitude and the harmonised diversity in Love, so that all relations of the play remain possible to us even while we retain on the heights of our being the eternal oneness with the Beloved. And by a similar wideness, being capable of a freedom in spirit that embraces life and does not depend upon withdrawal from life, we are able to become without egoism, bondage or reaction the channel in our mind and body for a divine action poured out freely upon the world.

The divine existence is of the nature not only of freedom, but of purity, beatitude and perfection. An integral purity which shall enable on the one hand the perfect reflection of the divine Being in ourselves and on the other the perfect outpouring of its Truth and Law in us in the terms of life and through the right functioning of the complex instrument we are in our outer parts, is the condition of an integral liberty. Its result is an integral beatitude, in which there becomes possible at once the Ananda of all that is in the world seen as symbols of the Divine and the Ananda of that which is not-world. And it prepares the integral perfection of our humanity as a type of the Divine in the conditions of the human manifestation, a perfection founded on a certain free universality of being, of love and joy, of play of knowledge and of play of will in power and will in unegoistic action. This integrality also can be attained by the integral Yoga.

Perfection includes perfection of mind and body, so that the highest results of Rajayoga and Hathayoga should be contained in the widest formula of the synthesis finally to be effected by mankind. At any rate a full development of the general mental and physical faculties and experiences attainable by humanity through Yoga must be included in the scope of the integral method. Nor would these have any *raison d'être* unless employed for an integral mental and physical life. Such a mental and physical life would be in its nature a translation of the spiritual existence into its right mental and physical values. Thus we would arrive at a synthesis of the three degrees of Nature and of the three modes of human existence which she has evolved or is evolving. We would include in the scope of our liberated being and perfected modes of activity the material life, our base, and the mental life, our intermediate instrument.

Nor would the integrality to which we aspire be real or even possible, if it were confined to the individual. Since our divine perfection embraces the realisation of ourselves in being, in life and in love through others as well as through ourselves, the extension of our liberty and of its results in others would be the inevitable outcome as well as the broadest utility of our liberation and perfection. And the constant and inherent attempt of such an extension would be towards its increasing and ultimately complete generalisation in mankind.

The divinising of the normal material life of man and of his great secular attempt of mental and moral self-culture in the individual and the race by this integralisation of a widely perfect spiritual existence would thus be the crown alike of our individual and of our common effort. Such a consummation being no other than the kingdom of heaven within reproduced in the kingdom of heaven without, would be also the true fulfilment of the great dream cherished in different terms by the world's religions.

The widest synthesis of perfection possible to thought is the sole effort entirely worthy of those whose dedicated vision perceives that God dwells concealed in humanity.

---

1. *Sādhana*, the practice by which perfection, *siddhi*, is attained; *sādhaka*, the Yogin who seeks by that practice the *siddhi*.
2. As the Jivanmukta, who is entirely free even without dissolution of the bodily life in a final Samadhi.

# THE YOGA OF INTEGRAL KNOWLEDGE

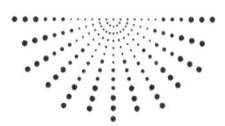

# THE OBJECT OF KNOWLEDGE

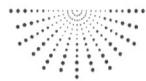

ALL SPIRITUAL seeking moves towards an object of Knowledge to which men ordinarily do not turn the eye of the mind, to someone or something Eternal, Infinite, Absolute that is not the temporal things or forces of which we are sensible, although he or it may be in them or behind them or their source or creator. It aims at a state of knowledge by which we can touch, enter or know by identity this Eternal, Infinite and Absolute, a consciousness other than our ordinary consciousness of ideas and forms and things, a Knowledge that is not what we call knowledge but something self-existent, everlasting, infinite. And although it may or even necessarily must, since man is a mental creature, start from our ordinary instruments of knowledge, yet it must as necessarily go beyond them and use supra-sensuous and supramental means and faculties, for it is in search of something that is itself supra-sensuous and supramental and beyond the grasp of the mind and senses, even if through mind and sense there can come a first glimpse of it or a reflected image.

The traditional systems, whatever their other differences, all proceed on the belief or the perception that the Eternal and Absolute can only be or at least can only inhabit a pure transcendent state of non-cosmic existence or else a non-existence. All cosmic existence or all that we call existence is a state of ignorance. Even the highest individual perfection, even the most blissful cosmic condition is no better than a supreme ignorance. All that is individual, all that is cosmic has to be austerely renounced by the seeker of the absolute Truth. The supreme quiescent Self or else the absolute Nihil is the sole Truth, the only object of spiritual knowledge. The state of knowledge, the consciousness other than this temporal that we must attain is Nirvana, an extinction of ego, a cessation of all mental, vital and physical activities, of all activities whatsoever, a supreme illumined quiescence, the pure bliss of an impersonal tranquillity self-absorbed and ineffable. The means are meditation, a concentration excluding all things else, a total loss of the mind in its object. Action is permissible only in the first stages of the search in order to purify the seeker and make him morally and temperamentally a fit vessel for the knowledge. Even this action must either be confined to the performance of the rites of worship and the prescribed duties of life rigorously ordained by the Hindu Shastra or, as in the Buddhistic discipline, must be guided along the eightfold path to the supreme practice of the works of compassion which lead towards the practical annihilation of self in the good of others. In the end, in any severe and pure Jnanayoga, all works must be abandoned for an entire quiescence. Action may prepare salvation; it cannot give it. Any continued adherence to action is incompatible with the highest progress and may be an insuperable obstacle to the attainment of the spiritual goal. The supreme state of quiescence is the very opposite of action and cannot be attained by those who persist in works. And even devotion, love, worship are disciplines for the unripe soul, are at best the best methods of the Ignorance. For they are offered to something other, higher and greater than ourselves; but in the supreme knowledge there can be no such thing, since there is either only one self or no self at all and therefore either no one to do the worship and offer the love and devotion or no one to receive it. Even thought-activity must disappear in the sole consciousness of identity or of nothingness and by its own quiescence bring about the quiescence of the whole nature. The absolute Identical alone must remain or else the eternal Nihil.

This pure Jnanayoga comes by the intellect, although it ends in the transcendence of the intellect and its workings. The thinker in us separates himself from all the rest of what we phenomenally are, rejects the heart, draws back from the life and the senses, separates from the body that he may arrive at his own exclusive fulfilment in that which is beyond even himself and his function. There is a truth that underlies, as there is an experience that seems to justify this attitude. There is an Essence that is in its nature a quiescence, a supreme of Silence in the Being that is beyond its own developments and mutations, immutable and therefore superior to all activities of which it is at most a Witness. And in the hierarchy of our psychological functions the Thought is in a way nearest to this Self, nearest at least to its aspect of the all-conscious knower who regards all activities but can stand back from them all. The heart, will and other powers in us are fundamentally active, turn naturally towards action, find through it their fulfilment,—although they also may automatically arrive at a certain quiescence by fullness of satisfaction in their activities or else by a reverse process of exhaustion through perpetual disappointment and dissatisfaction. The thought too is an active power, but is more capable of arriving at quiescence by its own conscious choice and will. The thought is more easily content with the illumined intellectual perception of this silent Witness Self that is higher than all our activities and, that immobile Spirit once seen, is ready, deeming its mission of truth-finding accomplished, to fall at rest and become itself immobile. For in its most characteristic movement it is itself apt to be a disinterested witness, judge, observer of things more than an eager participant and passionate labourer in the work and can arrive very readily at a spiritual or philosophic calm and detached aloofness. And since men are mental beings, thought, if not truly their best and highest, is at least their most constant, normal and effective means for enlightening their ignorance. Armed with its functions of gathering and reflection, meditation, fixed contemplation, the absorbed dwelling of the mind on its object, *śravaṇa, manana, nididhyāsana*, it stands at our tops as an indispensable aid to our realisation of that which we pursue, and it is not surprising that it should claim to be the leader of the journey and the only available guide or at least the direct and innermost door of the temple.

In reality, thought is only a scout and pioneer; it can guide but not command or effectuate. The leader of the journey, the captain of the march, the first and most ancient priest of our sacrifice is the Will. This Will is not the wish of the heart or the demand or preference of the mind to which we often give the name. It is that inmost, dominant and often veiled conscious force of our being and of all being, Tapas, Shakti, Sraddha, that sovereignly determines our orientation and of which the intellect and the heart are more or less blind and automatic servants and instruments. The Self that is quiescent, at rest, vacant of things and happenings is a support and background to existence, a silent channel or a hypostasis of something Supreme: it is not itself the one entirely real existence, not itself the Supreme. The Eternal, the Supreme is the Lord and the all-originating Spirit. Superior to all activities and not bound by any of them, it is the source, sanction, material, efficient power, master of all activities. All activities proceed from this supreme Self and are determined by it; all are its operations, processes of its own conscious force and not of something alien to Self, some power other than the Spirit. In these activities is expressed the conscious Will or Shakti of the Spirit moved to manifest its being in infinite ways, a Will or Power not ignorant but at one with its own self-knowledge and its knowledge of all that it is put out to express. And of this Power a secret spiritual will and soul-faith in us, the dominant hidden force of our nature, is the individual instrument, more nearly in communication with the Supreme, a surer guide and enlightener, could we once get at it and hold it, because profounder and more intimately near to the Identical and Absolute than the surface activities of our thought powers. To know that will in ourselves and in the universe and follow it to its divine finalities, whatever these may be, must surely be the highest way and truest culmination for knowledge as for works, for the seeker in life and for the seeker in Yoga.

The thought, since it is not the highest or strongest part of Nature, not even the sole or deepest index to Truth, ought not to follow its own exclusive satisfaction or take that for the sign of its attainment to the supreme Knowledge. It is here as the guide, up to a certain point, of the heart, the life and the other members, but it cannot be a substitute for them; it has to see not only what is its own ultimate satisfaction but whether there is not an ultimate satisfaction intended also for these other members. An exclusive path of abstract thought would be justified, only if the object of the Supreme Will in the universe has been nothing more than a descent into the activity of the ignorance operated by the mind as blinding instrument and jailor through false idea and sensation and an ascent into the quiescence of knowledge equally operated by the mind through correct thought as enlightening instrument and saviour. But the chances are that there is an aim in the world less absurd and aimless, an impulse towards the Absolute less dry and abstract, a truth of the world more large and complex, a more richly infinite height of the Infinite. Certainly, an abstract logic must always arrive, as the old systems arrived, at an infinite empty Negation or an infinite equally vacant Affirmation; for, abstract it moves towards an absolute abstraction and these are the only two abstractions that are absolutely absolute. But a concrete ever deepening wisdom waiting on more and more riches of infinite experience and not the confident abstract logic of the narrow and incompetent human mind is likely to be the key to a divine suprahuman knowledge. The heart, the will, the life and even the body, no less than the thought, are forms of a divine Conscious-Being and indices of great significance. These too have powers by which the soul can return to its complete self-awareness or means by which it can enjoy it. The object of the Supreme Will may well be a culmination in which the whole being is intended to receive its divine satisfaction, the heights enlightening the depths, the material Inconscient revealed to itself as the Divine by the touch of the supreme Superconscience.

The traditional Way of Knowledge proceeds by elimination and rejects successively the body, the life, the senses, the heart, the very thought in order to merge into the quiescent Self or supreme Nihil or indefinite Absolute. The way of integral knowledge supposes that we are intended to arrive at an integral self-fulfilment and the only thing that is to be eliminated is our own unconsciousness, the Ignorance and the results of the Ignorance. Eliminate the falsity of the being which figures as the ego; then our true being can manifest in us. Eliminate the falsity of the life which figures as mere vital craving and the mechanical round of our corporeal existence; our true life in the power of the Godhead and the joy of the Infinite will appear. Eliminate the falsity of the senses with their subjection to material shows and to dual sensations; there is a greater sense in us that can open through these to the Divine in things and divinely reply to it. Eliminate the falsity of the heart with its turbid passions and desires and its dual emotions; a deeper heart in us can open with its divine love for all creatures and its infinite passion and yearning for the responses of the Infinite. Eliminate the falsity of the thought with its imperfect mental constructions, its arrogant assertions and denials, its limited and exclusive concentrations; a greater faculty of knowledge is behind that can open to the true Truth of God and the soul and Nature and the universe. An integral self-fulfilment,—an absolute, a culmination for the experiences of the heart, for its instinct of love, joy, devotion and worship; an absolute, a culmination for the senses, for their pursuit of divine beauty and good and delight in the forms of things; an absolute, a culmination for the life, for its pursuit of works, of divine power, mastery and perfection; an absolute, a culmination beyond its own limits for the thought, for its hunger after truth and light and divine wisdom and knowledge. Not something quite other than themselves from which they are all cast away is the end of these things in our nature, but something supreme in which they at once transcend themselves and find their own absolutes and infinitudes, their harmonies beyond measure.

Behind the traditional way of Knowledge, justifying its thought-process of elimination and withdrawal, stands an overmastering spiritual experience. Deep, intense, convincing, common to all who have overstepped a certain limit of the active mind-belt into horizonless inner space, this is the great experience of liberation, the consciousness of something within us that is behind and outside of the universe and all its forms, interests, aims, events and happenings, calm, untouched, unconcerned, illimitable, immobile, free, the up-look to something above us indescribable and unseizable into which by abolition of our personality we can enter, the presence of an omnipresent eternal witness Purusha, the sense of an Infinity or a Timelessness that looks down on us from an august negation of all our existence and is alone the one thing Real. This experience is the highest sublimation of spiritualised mind looking resolutely beyond its own existence. No one who has not passed through this liberation can be entirely free from the mind and its meshes, but one is not compelled to linger in this experience for ever. Great as it is, it is only the Mind's overwhelming experience of what is beyond itself and all it can conceive. It is a supreme negative experience, but beyond it is all the tremendous light of an infinite Consciousness, an illimitable Knowledge, an affirmative absolute Presence.

The object of spiritual knowledge is the Supreme, the Divine, the Infinite and Absolute. This Supreme has its relations to our individual being and its relations to the universe and it transcends both the soul and the universe. Neither the universe nor the individual are what they seem to be, for the report of them which our mind and our senses give us is, so long as they are unenlightened by a faculty of higher supramental and suprasensuous knowledge, a false report, an imperfect construction, an attenuated and erroneous figure. And yet that which the universe and the individual seem to be is still a figure of what they really are, a figure that points beyond itself to the reality behind it. Truth proceeds by a correction of the values our mind and senses give us, and first by the action of a higher intelligence that enlightens and sets right as far as may be the conclusions of the ignorant sense-mind and limited physical intelligence; that is the method of all human knowledge and science. But beyond it there is a knowledge, a Truth-consciousness, that exceeds our intellect and brings us into the true light of which it is a refracted ray. There the abstract terms of the pure reason and the constructions of the mind disappear or are converted into concrete soul-vision and the tremendous actuality of spiritual experience. This knowledge can turn away to the absolute Eternal and lose vision of the soul and the universe; but it can too see this existence from that Eternal. When that is done, we find that the ignorance of the mind and the senses and all the apparent futilities of human life were not a useless excursion of the conscious being, an otiose blunder. Here they were planned as a rough ground for the self-expression of the Soul that comes from the Infinite, a material foundation for its self-unfolding and self-possessing in the terms of the universe. It is true that in themselves they and all that is here have no significance and to build separate significances for them is to live in an illusion, Maya; but they have a supreme significance in the Supreme, an absolute Power in the Absolute and it is that that assigns to them and refers to that Truth their present relative values. This is the all-uniting experience that is the foundation of the deepest integral and most intimate self-knowledge and world-knowledge.

In relation to the individual the Supreme is our own true and highest self, that which ultimately we are in our essence, that of which we are in our manifested nature. A spiritual knowledge, moved to arrive at the true Self in us, must reject, as the traditional way of knowledge rejects, all misleading appearances. It must discover that the body is not our self, our foundation of existence; it is a sensible form of the Infinite. The experience of Matter as the world's sole foundation and the physical brain and nerves and cells and molecules as the one truth of all things in us, the ponderous inadequate basis of materialism, is a delusion, a half-view taken for the whole, the dark bottom or shadow of things misconceived as the luminous substance, the effective figure of zero for the Integer. The materialist idea mistakes a creation for the creative Power, a means of expression for That which is expressed and expresses. Matter and our physical brain and nerves and body are the field and foundation for one action of a vital force that serves to connect the Self with the form of its works and maintains them by its direct dynamis. The material movements are an exterior notation by which the soul represents its perceptions of certain truths of the Infinite and makes them effective in the terms of Substance. These things are a language, a notation, a hieroglyphic, a system of symbols, not themselves the deepest truest sense of the things they intimate.

Neither is the Life ourself, the vitality, the energy which plays in the brain, nerves and body; it is a power and not the whole power of the Infinite. The experience of a life-force instrumentalising Matter as the foundation, source and true sum of all things, the vibrating unsteady basis of vitalism, is a delusion, a half-view taken for the whole, a tide on a near shore misconceived as all the ocean and its waters. The vitalist idea takes something powerful but outward for the essence. Life-force is the dynamisation of a consciousness which exceeds it. That consciousness is felt and acts but does not become valid to us in intelligence until we arrive at the higher term of Mind, our present summit. Mind is here apparently a creation of Life, but it is really the ulterior—not the ultimate —sense of Life itself and what is behind it and a more conscious formulation of its secret; Mind is an expression not of Life, but of that of which Life itself is a less luminous expression.

And yet Mind also, our mentality, our thinking, understanding part, is not our Self, is not That, not the end or the beginning; it is a half-light thrown from the Infinite. The experience of mind as the creator of forms and things and of these forms and things existing in the Mind only, the thin subtle basis of idealism, is also a delusion, a half-view taken for the whole, a pale refracted light idealised as the burning body of the Sun and its splendour. This idealist vision also does not arrive at the essence of being, does not even touch it but only an inferior mode of Nature. Mind is the dubious outer penumbra of a conscious existence which is not limited by mentality but exceeds it. The method of the traditional way of knowledge, eliminating all these things, arrives at the conception and realisation of a pure conscious existence, self-aware, self-blissful, unconditioned by mind and life and body and to its ultimate positive experience that is Atman, the Self, the original and essential nature of our existence. Here at last there is something centrally true, but in its haste to arrive at it this knowledge assumes that there is nothing between the thinking mind and the Highest, *buddheḥ paratas tu saḥ* , and, shutting its eyes in Samadhi, tries to rush through all that actually intervenes without even seeing these great and luminous kingdoms of the Spirit. Perhaps it arrives at its object, but only to fall asleep in the Infinite. Or, if it remains awake, it is in the highest experience of the Supreme into which the self-annulling Mind can enter, but not in the supreme of the Supreme, Paratpara. The Mind can only be aware of the Self in a mentalised spiritual thinness, only of the mind-reflected Sachchidananda. The highest truth, the integral self-knowledge is not to be gained by this self-blinded leap into the Absolute but by a patient transit beyond the mind into the Truth-consciousness where the Infinite can be known, felt, seen, experienced in all the fullness of its unending riches. And there we discover this Self that we are to be not only a static tenuous vacant Atman but a great dynamic Spirit individual, universal and transcendent. That Self and Spirit cannot be expressed by the mind's abstract generalisations; all the inspired descriptions of the seers and mystics cannot exhaust its contents and its splendours.

In relation to the universe the Supreme is Brahman, the one Reality which is not only the spiritual material and conscious substance of all the ideas and forces and forms of the universe, but their origin, support and possessor, the cosmic and supracosmic Spirit. All the last terms to which we can reduce the universe, Force and Matter, Name and Form, Purusha and Prakriti, are still not entirely that which the universe really is, either in itself or its nature. As all that we are is the play and form, the mental, psychic, vital and physical expression of a supreme Self unconditioned by mind and life and body, the universe too is the play and form and cosmic soul-expression and nature-expression of a supreme Existence which is unconditioned by force and matter, unconditioned by idea and name and form, unconditioned by the fundamental distinction of Purusha and Prakriti. Our supreme Self and the supreme Existence which has become the universe are one Spirit, one self and one existence. The individual is in nature one expression of the universal Being, in spirit an emanation of the Transcendence. For if he finds his self, he finds too that his own true self is not this natural personality, this created individuality, but is a universal being in its relations with others and with Nature and in its upward term a portion or the living front of a supreme transcendental Spirit.

This supreme Existence is not conditioned by the individual or by the universe. A spiritual knowledge can therefore surpass or even eliminate these two powers of the Spirit and arrive at the conception of something utterly Transcendent, something that is unnameable and mentally unknowable, a sheer Absolute. The traditional way of knowledge eliminates individual and universe. The Absolute it seeks after is featureless, indefinable, relationless, not this, not that, *neti neti*. And yet we can say of it that it is One, that it is Infinite, that it is ineffable Bliss, Consciousness, Existence. Although unknowable to the mind, yet through our individual being and through the names and forms of the universe we can approach the realisation of the supreme Self that is Brahman, and by the realisation of the self we come to a certain realisation also of this utter Absolute of which our true self is the essential form in our consciousness (*svarūpa*). These are the devices the human mind is compelled to use if it is to form to itself any conception at all of a transcendent and unconditioned Absolute. The system of negation is indispensable to it in order to get rid of its own definitions and limited experience; it is obliged to escape through a vague Indefinite into the Infinite. For it lives in a closed prison of constructions and representations that are necessary for its action but are not the self-existent truth either of Matter or Life or Mind or Spirit. But if we can once cross beyond the Mind's frontier twilight into the vast plane of supramental Knowledge, these devices cease to be indispensable. Supermind has quite another, a positive and direct and living experience of the supreme Infinite. The Absolute is beyond personality and beyond impersonality, and yet it is both the Impersonal and the supreme Person and all persons. The Absolute is beyond the distinction of unity and multiplicity, and yet it is the One and the innumerable Many in all the universes. It is beyond all limitation by quality and yet it is not limited by a qualitiless void but is too all infinite qualities. It is the individual soul and all souls and none of them; it is the formless Brahman and the universe. It is the cosmic and the supracosmic Spirit, the supreme Lord, the supreme Self, the supreme Purusha and supreme Shakti, the Ever Unborn who is endlessly born, the Infinite who is innumerably finite, the multitudinous One, the complex Simple, the many-sided Single, the Word of the Silence Ineffable, the impersonal omnipresent Person, the Mystery translucent in highest consciousness to its own spirit, but to a lesser consciousness veiled in its own exceeding light and impenetrable for ever. These things are to the dimensional mind irreconcilable opposites, but to the constant vision and experience of the supramental Truth-consciousness they are so simply and inevitably the intrinsic nature of each other that even to think of them as contraries is an unimaginable violence. The walls constructed by the measuring and separating Intellect have disappeared and the Truth in its simplicity and beauty appears and reduces all to terms of its harmony and unity and light. Dimensions and distinctions remain but as figures for use, not a separative prison for the self-forgetting Spirit.

The consciousness of the transcendent Absolute with its consequence in individual and universe is the last, the eternal knowledge. Our minds may deal with it on various lines, may build upon it conflicting philosophies, may limit, modify, overstress, understress sides of the knowledge, deduce from it truth or error; but our intellectual variations and imperfect statements make no difference to the ultimate fact that if we push thought and experience to their end, this is the knowledge in which they terminate. The object of a Yoga of spiritual knowledge can be nothing else than this eternal Reality, this Self, this Brahman, this Transcendent that dwells over all and in all and is manifest yet concealed in the individual, manifest yet disguised in the universe.

The culmination of the path of knowledge need not necessarily entail extinction of our world-existence. For the Supreme to whom we assimilate ourselves, the Absolute and Transcendent into whom we enter has always the complete and ultimate consciousness for which we are seeking and yet he supports by it his play in the world. Neither are we compelled to believe that our world-existence ends because by attaining to knowledge its object or consummation is fulfilled and therefore there is nothing more for us here afterwards. For what we gain at first with its release and immeasurable silence and quietude is only the eternal self-realisation by the individual in the essence of his conscious being; there will still remain on that foundation, unannulled by the silence, one with the release and freedom, the infinitely proceeding self-fulfilment of Brahman, its dynamic divine manifestation in the individual and by his presence, example and action in others and in the universe at large,—the work which the Great Ones remain to do. Our dynamic self-fulfilment cannot be worked out so long as we remain in the egoistic consciousness, in the mind's candle-lit darkness, in the bondage. Our present limited consciousness can only be a field of preparation, it can consummate nothing; for all that it manifests is marred through and through by an ego-ridden ignorance and error. The true and divine self-fulfilment of Brahman in the manifestation is only possible on the foundation of the Brahman-consciousness and therefore through the acceptance of life by the liberated soul, the Jivanmukta.

This is the integral knowledge; for we know that everywhere and in all conditions all to the eye that sees is One, to a divine experience all is one block of the Divine. It is only the mind which for the temporary convenience of its own thought and aspiration seeks to cut an artificial line of rigid division, a fiction of perpetual incompatibility between one aspect and another of the eternal oneness. The liberated knower lives and acts in the world not less than the bound soul and ignorant mind but more, doing all actions, *sarvakṛt*, only with a true knowledge and a greater conscient power. And by so doing he does not forfeit the supreme unity nor fall from the supreme consciousness and the highest knowledge. For the Supreme, however hidden now to us, is here in the world no less than he could be in the most utter and ineffable self-extinction, the most intolerant Nirvana.

# THE STATUS OF KNOWLEDGE

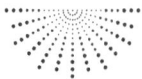

THE SELF, the Divine, the Supreme Reality, the All, the Transcendent,—the One in all these aspects is then the object of Yogic knowledge. Ordinary objects, the external appearances of life and matter, the psychology of our thoughts and actions, the perception of the forces of the apparent world can be part of this knowledge, but only in so far as it is part of the manifestation of the One. It becomes at once evident that the knowledge for which Yoga strives must be different from what men ordinarily understand by the word. For we mean ordinarily by knowledge an intellectual appreciation of the facts of life, mind and matter and the laws that govern them. This is a knowledge founded upon our sense-perception and upon reasoning from our sense-perceptions and it is undertaken partly for the pure satisfaction of the intellect, partly for practical efficiency and the added power which knowledge gives in managing our lives and the lives of others, in utilising for human ends the overt or secret forces of Nature and in helping or hurting, in saving and ennobling or in oppressing and destroying our fellow-men. Yoga, indeed, is commensurate with all life and can include all these subjects and objects. There is even a Yoga[1] which can be used for self-indulgence as well as for self-conquest, for hurting others as well as for their salvation. But "all life" includes not only, not even mainly life as humanity now leads it. It envisages rather and regards as its one true object a higher truly conscious existence which our half-conscious humanity does not yet possess and can only arrive at by a self-exceeding spiritual ascension. It is this greater consciousness and higher existence which is the peculiar and appropriate object of Yogic discipline. This greater consciousness, this higher existence are not an enlightened or illumined mentality supported by a greater dynamic energy or supporting a purer moral life and character. Their superiority to the ordinary human consciousness is not in degree but in kind and essence. There is a change not merely of the surface or instrumental manner of our being but of its very foundation and dynamic principle. Yogic knowledge seeks to enter into a secret consciousness beyond mind which is only occultly here, concealed at the basis of all existence. For it is that consciousness alone that truly knows and only by its possession can we possess God and rightly know the world and its real nature and secret forces. All this world visible or sensible to us and all too in it that is not visible is merely the phenomenal expression of something beyond the mind and the senses. The knowledge which the senses and intellectual reasoning from the data of the senses can bring us, is not true knowledge; it is a science of appearances. And even appearances cannot be properly known unless we know first the Reality of which they are images. This Reality is their self and there is one self of all; when that is seized, all other things can then be known in their truth and no longer as now only in their appearance.

It is evident that however much we may analyse the physical and sensible, we cannot by that means arrive at the knowledge of the Self or of ourselves or of that which we call God. The telescope, the microscope, the scalpel, the retort and alembic cannot go beyond the physical, although they may arrive at subtler and subtler truths about the physical. If then we confine ourselves to what the senses and their physical aids reveal to us and refuse from the beginning to admit any other reality or any other means of knowledge, we are obliged to conclude that nothing is real except the physical and that there is no Self in us or in the universe, no God within and without, no ourselves even except this aggregate of brain, nerves and body. But this we are only obliged to conclude because we have assumed it firmly from the beginning and therefore cannot but circle round to our original assumption.

If, then, there is a Self, a Reality not obvious to the senses, it must be by other means than those of physical Science that it is to be sought and known. The intellect is not that means. Undoubtedly there are a number of suprasensuous truths at which the intellect is able to arrive in its own manner and which it is able to perceive and state as intellectual conceptions. The very idea of Force for instance on which Science so much insists, is a conception, a truth at which the intellect alone can arrive by going beyond its data; for we do not sense this universal force but only its results, and the force itself we infer as a necessary cause of these results. So also the intellect by following a certain line of rigorous analysis can arrive at the intellectual conception and the intellectual conviction of the Self and this conviction can be very real, very luminous, very potent as the beginning of other and greater things. Still, in itself intellectual analysis can only lead to an arrangement of clear conceptions, perhaps to a right arrangement of true conceptions; but this is not the knowledge aimed at by Yoga. For it is not in itself an effective knowledge. A man may be perfect in it and yet be precisely what he was before except in the mere fact of the greater intellectual illumination. The change of our being at which Yoga aims, may not at all take place.

It is true that intellectual deliberation and right discrimination are an important part of the Yoga of knowledge; but their object is rather to remove a difficulty than to arrive at the final and positive result of this path. Our ordinary intellectual notions are a stumbling-block in the way of knowledge; for they are governed by the error of the senses and they found themselves on the notion that matter and body are the reality, that life and force are the reality, that passion and emotion, thought and sense are the reality; and with these things we identify ourselves, and because we identify ourselves with these things we cannot get back to the real self. Therefore, it is necessary for the seeker of knowledge to remove this stumbling-block and to get right notions about himself and the world; for how shall we pursue by knowledge the real self if we have no notion of what it is and are on the contrary burdened with ideas quite opposite to the truth?

Therefore right thought is a necessary preliminary, and once the habit of right thought is established, free from sense-error and desire and old association and intellectual prejudgment, the understanding becomes purified and offers no serious obstacle to the farther process of knowledge. Still, right thought only becomes effective when in the purified understanding it is followed by other operations, by vision, by experience, by realisation.

What are these operations? They are not mere psychological self-analysis and self-observation. Such analysis, such observation are, like the process of right thought, of immense value and practically indispensable. They may even, if rightly pursued, lead to a right thought of considerable power and effectivity. Like intellectual discrimination by the process of meditative thought they will have an effect of purification; they will lead to self-knowledge of a certain kind and to the setting right of the disorders of the soul and the heart and even of the disorders of the understanding. Self-knowledge of all kinds is on the straight path to the knowledge of the real Self. The Upanishad tells us that the Self-existent has so set the doors of the soul that they turn outwards and most men look outward into the appearances of things; only the rare soul that is ripe for a calm thought and steady wisdom turns its eye inward, sees the Self and attains to immortality. To this turning of the eye inward psychological self-observation and analysis is a great and effective introduction. We can look into the inward of ourselves more easily than we can look into the inward of things external to us because there, in things outside us, we are in the first place embarrassed by the form and secondly we have no natural previous experience of that in them which is other than their physical substance. A purified or tranquillised mind may reflect or a powerful concentration may discover God in the world, the Self in Nature even before it is realised in ourselves, but this is rare and difficult.[2] And it is only in ourselves that we can observe and know the process of the Self in its becoming and follow the process by which it draws back into self-being. Therefore the ancient counsel, know thyself, will always stand as the first word that directs us towards *the* knowledge. Still, psychological self-knowledge is only the experience of the modes of the Self, it is not the realisation of the Self in its pure being.

The status of knowledge, then, which Yoga envisages is not merely an intellectual conception or clear discrimination of the truth, nor is it an enlightened psychological experience of the modes of our being. It is a "realisation", in the full sense of the word; it is the making real to ourselves and in ourselves of the Self, the transcendent and universal Divine, and it is the subsequent impossibility of viewing the modes of being except in the light of that Self and in their true aspect as its flux of becoming under the psychical and physical conditions of our world-existence. This realisation consists of three successive movements, internal vision, complete internal experience and identity.

This internal vision, *dṛṣṭi*, the power so highly valued by the ancient sages, the power which made a man a Rishi or Kavi and no longer a mere thinker, is a sort of light in the soul by which things unseen become as evident and real to it—to the soul and not merely to the intellect—as do things seen to the physical eye. In the physical world there are always two forms of knowledge, the direct and the indirect, *pratyakṣa*, of that which is present to the eyes, and *parokṣa*, of that which is remote from and beyond our vision. When the object is beyond our vision, we are necessarily obliged to arrive at an idea of it by inference, imagination, analogy, by hearing the descriptions of others who have seen it or by studying pictorial or other representations of it if these are available. By putting together all these aids we can indeed arrive at a more or less adequate idea or suggestive image of the object, but we do not realise the thing itself; it is not yet to us the grasped reality, but only our conceptual representation of a reality. But once we have seen it with the eyes,—for no other sense is adequate,—we possess, we realise; it is there secure in our satisfied being, part of ourselves in knowledge.

Precisely the same rule holds good of psychical things and of the Self. We may hear clear and luminous teachings about the Self from philosophers or teachers or from ancient writings; we may by thought, inference, imagination, analogy or by any other available means attempt to form a mental figure or conception of it; we may hold firmly that conception in our mind and fix it by an entire and exclusive concentration;[3] but we have not yet realised it, we have not seen God. It is only when after long and persistent concentration or by other means the veil of the mind is rent or swept aside, only when a flood of light breaks over the awakened mentality, *jyotirmaya brahman*, and conception gives place to a knowledge-vision in which the Self is as present, real, concrete as a physical object to the physical eye, that we possess in knowledge; for we have seen. After that revelation, whatever fadings of the light, whatever periods of darkness may afflict the soul, it can never irretrievably lose what it has once held. The experience is inevitably renewed and must become more frequent till it is constant; when and how soon depends on the devotion and persistence with which we insist on the path and besiege by our will or our love the hidden Deity.

This inner vision is one form of psychological experience; but the inner experience is not confined to that seeing; vision only opens, it does not embrace. Just as the eye, though it is alone adequate to bring the first sense of realisation, has to call in the aid of experience by the touch and other organs of sense before there is an embracing knowledge, so the vision of the self ought to be completed by an experience of it in all our members. Our whole being ought to demand God and not only our illumined eye of knowledge.

For since each principle in us is only a manifestation of the Self, each can get back to its reality and have the experience of it. We can have a mental experience of the Self and seize as concrete realities all those apparently abstract things that to the mind constitute existence—consciousness, force, delight and their manifold forms and workings: thus the mind is satisfied of God. We can have an emotional experience of the Self through Love and through emotional delight, love and delight of the Self in us, of the Self in the universal and of the Self in all with whom we have relations: thus the heart is satisfied of God. We can have an aesthetic experience of the Self in beauty, a delight-perception and taste of the absolute reality all-beautiful in everything whether created by ourselves or Nature in its appeal to the aesthetic mind and the senses; thus the sense is satisfied of God. We can have even the vital, nervous experience and practically the physical sense of the Self in all life and formation and in all workings of powers, forces, energies that operate through us or others or in the world: thus the life and the body are satisfied of God.

All this knowledge and experience are primary means of arriving at and of possessing identity. It is our self that we see and experience and therefore vision and experience are incomplete unless they culminate in identity, unless we are able to live in all our being the supreme Vedantic knowledge, He am I. We must not only see God and embrace Him, but become that Reality. We must become one with the Self in its transcendence of all form and manifestation by the resolution, the sublimation, the escape from itself of ego and all its belongings into That from which they proceed, as well as become the Self in all its manifested existences and becomings, one with it in the infinite existence, consciousness, peace, delight by which it reveals itself in us and one with it in the action, formation, play of self-conception with which it garbs itself in the world.

It is difficult for the modern mind to understand how we can do more than conceive intellectually of the Self or of God; but it may borrow some shadow of this vision, experience and becoming from that inner awakening to Nature which a great English poet has made a reality to the European imagination. If we read the poems in which Wordsworth expressed his realisation of Nature, we may acquire some distant idea of what realisation is. For, first, we see that he had the vision of something in the world which is the very Self of all things that it contains, a conscious force and presence other than its forms, yet cause of its forms and manifested in them. We perceive that he had not only the vision of this and the joy and peace and universality which its presence brings, but the very sense of it, mental, aesthetic, vital, physical; not only this sense and vision of it in its own being but in the nearest flower and simplest man and the immobile rock; and, finally, that he even occasionally attained to that unity, that becoming the object of his meditation, one phase of which is powerfully and profoundly expressed in the poem "A slumber did my spirit seal," where he describes himself as become one in his being with earth, "rolled round in its diurnal course with rocks and stones and trees." Exalt this realisation to a profounder Self than physical Nature and we have the elements of the Yogic knowledge. But all this experience is only the vestibule to that suprasensuous, supramental realisation of the Transcendent who is beyond all His aspects, and the final summit of knowledge can only be attained by entering into the superconscient and there merging all other experience into a supernal unity with the Ineffable. That is the culmination of all divine knowing; that also is the source of all divine delight and divine living.

That status of knowledge is then the aim of this path and indeed of all paths when pursued to their end, to which intellectual discrimination and conception and all concentration and psychological self-knowledge and all seeking by the heart through love and by the senses through beauty and by the will through power and works and by the soul through peace and joy are only keys, avenues, first approaches and beginnings of the ascent which we have to use and to follow till the wide and infinite levels are attained and the divine doors swing open into the infinite Light.

---

1. Yoga develops power, it develops it even when we do not desire or consciously aim at it; and power is always a double-edged weapon which can be used to hurt or destroy as well as to help and save. Be it also noted that all destruction is not evil.
2. In one respect, however, it is easier, because in external things we are not so much hampered by the sense of the limited ego as in ourselves; one obstacle to the realisation of God is therefore removed.
3. This is the idea of the triple operation of Jnanayoga, *śravaṇa, manana, nididhyāsana*, hearing, thinking or mentalising and fixing in concentration.

# THE PURIFIED UNDERSTANDING

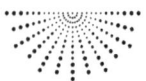

THE DESCRIPTION of the status of knowledge to which we aspire, determines the means of knowledge which we shall use. That status of knowledge may be summed up as a supramental realisation which is prepared by mental representations through various mental principles in us and once attained again reflects itself more perfectly in all the members of the being. It is a re-seeing and therefore a remoulding of our whole existence in the light of the Divine and One and Eternal free from subjection to the appearances of things and the externalities of our superficial being.

Such a passage from the human to the divine, from the divided and discordant to the One, from the phenomenon to the eternal Truth, such an entire rebirth or new birth of the soul must necessarily involve two stages, one of preparation in which the soul and its instruments must become fit and another of actual illumination and realisation in the prepared soul through its fit instruments. There is indeed no rigid line of demarcation in sequence of Time between these two stages; rather they are necessary to each other and continue simultaneously. For in proportion as the soul becomes fit it increases in illumination and rises to higher and higher, completer and completer realisations, and in proportion as these illuminations and these realisations increase, becomes fit and its instruments more adequate to their task: there are soul-seasons of unillumined preparation and soul-seasons of illumined growth and culminating soul-moments more or less prolonged of illumined possession, moments that are transient like the flash of the lightning, yet change the whole spiritual future, moments also that extend over many human hours, days, weeks in a constant light or blaze of the Sun of Truth. And through all these the soul once turned Godwards grows towards the permanence and perfection of its new birth and real existence.

The first necessity of preparation is the purifying of all the members of our being; especially, for the path of knowledge, the purification of the understanding, the key that shall open the door of Truth; and a purified understanding is hardly possible without the purification of the other members. An unpurified heart, an unpurified sense, an unpurified life confuse the understanding, disturb its data, distort its conclusions, darken its seeing, misapply its knowledge; an unpurified physical system clogs or chokes up its action. There must be an integral purity. Here also there is an interdependence; for the purification of each member of our being profits by the clarifying of every other, the progressive tranquillisation of the emotional heart helping for instance the purification of the understanding while equally a purified understanding imposes calm and light on the turbid and darkened workings of the yet impure emotions. It may even be said that while each member of our being has its own proper principles of purification, yet it is the purified understanding that in man is the most potent cleanser of his turbid and disordered being and most sovereignly imposes their right working on his other members. Knowledge, says the Gita, is the sovereign purity; light is the source of all clearness and harmony even as the darkness of ignorance is the cause of all our stumblings. Love, for example, is the purifier of the heart and by reducing all our emotions into terms of divine love the heart is perfected and fulfilled; yet love itself needs to be clarified by divine knowledge. The heart's love of God may be blind, narrow and ignorant and lead to fanaticism and obscurantism; it may, even when otherwise pure, limit our perfection by refusing to see Him except in a limited personality and by recoiling from the true and infinite vision. The heart's love of man may equally lead to distortions and exaggerations in feeling, action and knowledge which have to be corrected and prevented by the purification of the understanding.

We must, however, consider deeply and clearly what we mean by the understanding and by its purification. We use the word as the nearest equivalent we can get in the English tongue to the Sanskrit philosophical term *buddhi*; therefore we exclude from it the action of the sense mind which merely consists of the recording of perceptions of all kinds without distinction whether they be right or wrong, true or mere illusory phenomena, penetrating or superficial. We exclude that mass of confused conception which is merely a rendering of these perceptions and is equally void of the higher principle of judgment and discrimination. Nor can we include that constant leaping current of habitual thought which does duty for understanding in the mind of the average unthinking man, but is only a constant repetition of habitual associations, desires, prejudices, prejudgments, received or inherited preferences, even though it may constantly enrich itself by a fresh stock of concepts streaming in from the environment and admitted without the challenge of the sovereign discriminating reason. Undoubtedly this is a sort of understanding which has been very useful in the development of man from the animal; but it is only one remove above the animal mind; it is a half-animal reason subservient to habit, to desire and the senses and is of no avail in the search whether for scientific or philosophical or spiritual knowledge. We have to go beyond it; its purification can only be effected either by dismissing or silencing it altogether or by transmuting it into the true understanding.

By the understanding we mean that which at once perceives, judges and discriminates, the true reason of the human being not subservient to the senses, to desire or to the blind force of habit, but working in its own right for mastery, for knowledge. Certainly, the reason of man as he is at present does not even at its best act entirely in this free and sovereign fashion; but so far as it fails, it fails because it is still mixed with the lower half-animal action, because it is impure and constantly hampered and pulled down from its characteristic action. In its purity it should not be involved in these lower movements, but stand back from the object, and observe disinterestedly, put it in its right place in the whole by force of comparison, contrast, analogy, reason from its rightly observed data by deduction, induction, inference and holding all its gains in memory and supplementing them by a chastened and rightly-guided imagination view all in the light of a trained and disciplined judgment. Such is the pure intellectual understanding of which disinterested observation, judgment and reasoning are the law and characterising action.

But the term *buddhi* is also used in another and profounder sense. The intellectual understanding is only the lower *buddhi*; there is another and a higher *buddhi* which is not intelligence but vision, is not understanding but rather an over-standing[1] in knowledge, and does not seek knowledge and attain it in subjection to the data it observes but possesses already the truth and brings it out in the terms of a revelatory and intuitional thought. The nearest the human mind usually gets to this truth-conscious knowledge is that imperfect action of illumined finding which occurs when there is a great stress of thought and the intellect electrified by constant discharges from behind the veil and yielding to a higher enthusiasm admits a considerable instreaming from the intuitive and inspired faculty of knowledge. For there is an intuitive mind in man which serves as a recipient and channel for these instreamings from a supramental faculty. But the action of intuition and inspiration in us is imperfect in kind as well as intermittent in action; ordinarily, it comes in response to a claim from the labouring and struggling heart or intellect and, even before its givings enter the conscious mind, they are already affected by the thought or aspiration which went up to meet them, are no longer pure but altered to the needs of the heart or intellect; and after they enter the conscious mind, they are immediately seized upon by the intellectual understanding and dissipated or broken up so as to fit in with our imperfect intellectual knowledge, or by the heart and remoulded to suit our blind or half-blind emotional longings and preferences, or even by the lower cravings and distorted to the vehement uses of our hungers and passions.

If this higher *buddhi* could act pure of the interference of these lower members, it would give pure forms of the truth; observation would be dominated or replaced by a vision which could see without subservient dependence on the testimony of the sense-mind and senses; imagination would give place to the self-assured inspiration of the truth, reasoning to the spontaneous discernment of relations and conclusion from reasoning to an intuition containing in itself those relations and not building laboriously upon them, judgment to a thought-vision in whose light the truth would stand revealed without the mask which it now wears and which our intellectual judgment has to penetrate; while memory too would take upon itself that larger sense given to it in Greek thought and be no longer a paltry selection from the store gained by the individual in his present life, but rather the all-recording knowledge which secretly holds and constantly gives from itself everything that we now seem painfully to acquire but really in this sense remember, a knowledge which includes the future[2] no less than the past. Certainly, we are intended to grow in our receptivity to this higher faculty of truth-conscious knowledge, but its full and unveiled use is as yet the privilege of the gods and beyond our present human stature.

We see then what we mean precisely by the understanding and by that higher faculty which we may call for the sake of convenience the ideal faculty and which stands to the developed intellect much in the same relation as that intellect stands to the half-animal reason of the undeveloped man. It becomes evident also what is the nature of the purification which is necessary before the understanding can fulfil rightly its part in the attainment of right knowledge. All impurity is a confusion of working, a departure from the *dharma*, the just and inherently right action of things which in that right action are pure and helpful to our perfection and this departure is usually the result of an ignorant confusion[3] of dharmas in which the function lends itself to the demand of other tendencies than those which are properly its own.

The first cause of impurity in the understanding is the intermiscence of desire in the thinking functions, and desire itself is an impurity of the Will involved in the vital and emotional parts of our being. When the vital and emotional desires interfere with the pure will-to-know, the thought-function becomes subservient to them, pursues ends other than those proper to itself and its perceptions are clogged and deranged. The understanding must lift itself beyond the siege of desire and emotion and, in order that it may have perfect immunity, it must get the vital parts and the emotions themselves purified. The will to enjoy is proper to the vital being but not the choice or the reaching after the enjoyment which must be determined and acquired by higher functions; therefore the vital being must be trained to accept whatever gain or enjoyment comes to it in the right functioning of the life in obedience to the working of the divine Will and to rid itself of craving and attachment. Similarly the heart must be free from subjection to the cravings of the life-principle and the senses and thus rid itself of the false emotions of fear, wrath, hatred, lust, etc. which constitute the chief impurity of the heart. The will to love is proper to the heart, but here also the choice and reaching after love have to be foregone or tranquillised and the heart taught to love with depth and intensity indeed, but with a calm depth and a settled and equal, not a troubled and disordered intensity. The tranquillisation and mastery[4] of these members is a first condition for the immunity of the understanding from error, ignorance and perversion. This purification spells an entire equality of the nervous being and the heart; equality, therefore, even as it was the first word of the path of works, so also is the first word of the path of knowledge.

The second cause of impurity in the understanding is the illusion of the senses and the intermiscence of the sense-mind in the thinking functions. No knowledge can be true knowledge which subjects itself to the senses or uses them otherwise than as first indices whose data have constantly to be corrected and over-passed. The beginning of Science is the examination of the truths of the world-force that underlie its apparent workings such as our senses represent them to be; the beginning of philosophy is the examination of the principles of things which the senses mistranslate to us; the beginning of spiritual knowledge is the refusal to accept the limitations of the sense-life or to take the visible and sensible as anything more than phenomenon of the Reality.

Equally must the sense-mind be stilled and taught to leave the function of thought to the mind that judges and understands. When the understanding in us stands back from the action of the sense-mind and repels its intermiscence, the latter detaches itself from the understanding and can be watched in its separate action. It then reveals itself as a constantly swirling and eddying undercurrent of habitual concepts, associations, perceptions, desires without any real sequence, order or principle of light. It is a constant repetition in a circle unintelligent and unfruitful. Ordinarily the human understanding accepts this undercurrent and tries to reduce it to a partial order and sequence; but by so doing it becomes itself subject to it and partakes of that disorder, restlessness, unintelligent subjection to habit and blind purposeless repetition which makes the ordinary human reason a misleading, limited and even frivolous and futile instrument. There is nothing to be done with this fickle, restless, violent and disturbing factor but to get rid of it whether by detaching it and then reducing it to stillness or by giving a concentration and singleness to the thought by which it will of itself reject this alien and confusing element.

A third cause of impurity has its source in the understanding itself and consists in an improper action of the will to know. That will is proper to the understanding, but here again choice and unequal reaching after knowledge clog and distort. They lead to a partiality and attachment which makes the intellect cling to certain ideas and opinions with a more or less obstinate will to ignore the truth in other ideas and opinions, cling to certain fragments of a truth and shy against the admission of other parts which are yet necessary to its fullness, cling to certain predilections of knowledge and repel all knowledge that does not agree with the personal temperament of thought which has been acquired by the past of the thinker. The remedy lies in a perfect equality of the mind, in the cultivation of an entire intellectual rectitude and in the perfection of mental disinterestedness. The purified understanding as it will not lend itself to any desire or craving, so will not lend itself either to any predilection or distaste for any particular idea or truth, and will refuse to be attached even to those ideas of which it is the most certain or to lay on them such an undue stress as is likely to disturb the balance of truth and depreciate the values of other elements of a complete and perfect knowledge.

An understanding thus purified would be a perfectly flexible, entire and faultless instrument of intellectual thought and being free from the inferior sources of obstruction and distortion would be capable of as true and complete a perception of the truths of the Self and the universe as the intellect can attain. But for real knowledge something more is necessary, since real knowledge is by our very definition of it supra-intellectual. In order that the understanding may not interfere with our attainment to real knowledge, we have to reach to that something more and cultivate a power exceedingly difficult for the active intellectual thinker and distasteful to his proclivities, the power of intellectual passivity. The object served is double and therefore two different kinds of passivity have to be acquired.

In the first place we have seen that intellectual thought is in itself inadequate and is not the highest thinking; the highest is that which comes through the intuitive mind and from the supramental faculty. So long as we are dominated by the intellectual habit and by the lower workings, the intuitive mind can only send its messages to us subconsciously and subject to a distortion more or less entire before it reaches the conscious mind; or if it works consciously, then only with an inadequate rarity and a great imperfection in its functioning. In order to strengthen the higher knowledge-faculty in us we have to effect the same separation between the intuitive and intellectual elements of our thought as we have already effected between the understanding and the sense-mind; and this is no easy task, for not only do our intuitions come to us incrusted in the intellectual action, but there are a great number of mental workings which masquerade and ape the appearances of the higher faculty. The remedy is to train first the intellect to recognise the true intuition, to distinguish it from the false and then to accustom it, when it arrives at an intellectual perception or conclusion, to attach no final value to it, but rather look upward, refer all to the divine principle and wait in as complete a silence as it can command for the light from above. In this way it is possible to transmute a great part of our intellectual thinking into the luminous truth-conscious vision,—the ideal would be a complete transition,—or at least to increase greatly the frequency, purity and conscious force of the ideal knowledge working behind the intellect. The latter must learn to be subject and passive to the ideal faculty.

But for the knowledge of the Self it is necessary to have the power of a complete intellectual passivity, the power of dismissing all thought, the power of the mind to think not at all which the Gita in one passage enjoins. This is a hard saying for the occidental mind to which thought is the highest thing and which will be apt to mistake the power of the mind not to think, its complete silence for the incapacity of thought. But this power of silence is a capacity and not an incapacity, a power and not a weakness. It is a profound and pregnant stillness. Only when the mind is thus entirely still, like clear, motionless and level water, in a perfect purity and peace of the whole being and the soul transcends thought, can the Self which exceeds and originates all activities and becomings, the Silence from which all words are born, the Absolute of which all relativities are partial reflections manifest itself in the pure essence of our being. In a complete silence only is the Silence heard; in a pure peace only is its Being revealed. Therefore to us the name of That is the Silence and the Peace.

---

1. The Divine Being is described as the *adhyakṣa*, he who seated overall in the supreme ether over-sees things, views and controls them from above.
2. In this sense the power of prophecy has been aptly called a memory of the future.
3. *saṅkara*.
4. *śama* and *dama*.

# CONCENTRATION

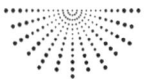

ALONG with purity and as a help to bring it about, concentration. Purity and concentration are indeed two aspects, feminine and masculine, passive and active, of the same status of being; purity is the condition in which concentration becomes entire, rightly effective, omnipotent; by concentration purity does its works and without it would only lead to a state of peaceful quiescence and eternal repose. Their opposites are also closely connected; for we have seen that impurity is a confusion of dharmas, a lax, mixed and mutually entangled action of the different parts of the being; and this confusion proceeds from an absence of right concentration of its knowledge on its energies in the embodied Soul. The fault of our nature is first an inert subjection to the impacts of things[1] as they come in upon the mind pell-mell without order or control and then a haphazard imperfect concentration managed fitfully, irregularly with a more or less chance emphasis on this or on that object according as they happen to interest, not the higher soul or the judging and discerning intellect, but the restless, leaping, fickle, easily tired, easily distracted lower mind which is the chief enemy of our progress. In such a condition purity, the right working of the functions, the clear, unstained and luminous order of the being is an impossibility; the various workings, given over to the chances of the environment and external influences, must necessarily run into each other and clog, divert, distract, pervert. Equally, without purity the complete, equal, flexible concentration of the being in right thought, right will, right feeling or secure status of spiritual experience is not possible. Therefore the two must proceed together, each helping the victory of the other, until we arrive at that eternal calm from which may proceed some partial image in the human being of the eternal, omnipotent and omniscient activity.

But in the path of knowledge as it is practised in India concentration is used in a special and more limited sense. It means that removal of the thought from all distracting activities of the mind and that concentration of it on the idea of the One by which the soul rises out of the phenomenal into the one Reality. It is by the thought that we dissipate ourselves in the phenomenal; it is by the gathering back of the thought into itself that we must draw ourselves back into the real. Concentration has three powers by which this aim can be effected. By concentration on anything whatsoever we are able to know that thing, to make it deliver up its concealed secrets; we must use this power to know not things, but the one Thing-in-itself. By concentration again the whole will can be gathered up for the acquisition of that which is still ungrasped, still beyond us; this power, if it is sufficiently trained, sufficiently single-minded, sufficiently sincere, sure of itself, faithful to itself alone, absolute in faith, we can use for the acquisition of any object whatsoever; but we ought to use it not for the acquisition of the many objects which the world offers to us, but to grasp spiritually that one object worthy of pursuit which is also the one subject worthy of knowledge. By concentration of our whole being on one status of itself, we can become whatever we choose; we can become, for instance, even if we were before a mass of weaknesses and fears, a mass instead of strength and courage, or we can become all a great purity, holiness and peace or a single universal soul of Love; but we ought, it is said, to use this power to become not even these things, high as they may be in comparison with what we now are, but rather to become that which is above all things and free from all action and attributes, the pure and absolute Being. All else, all other concentration can only be valuable for preparation, for previous steps, for a gradual training of the dissolute and self-dissipating thought, will and being towards their grand and unique object.

This use of concentration implies like every other a previous purification; it implies also in the end a renunciation, a cessation and lastly an ascent into the absolute and transcendent state of Samadhi from which if it culminates, if it endures, there is, except perhaps for one soul out of many thousands, no return. For by that we go to the "supreme state of the Eternal whence souls revert not" into the cyclic action of Nature;[2] and it is into this Samadhi that the Yogin who aims at release from the world seeks to pass away at the time of leaving his body. We see this succession in the discipline of the Rajayoga. For first the Rajayogin must arrive at a certain moral and spiritual purity; he must get rid of the lower or downward activities of his mind, but afterwards he must stop all its activities and concentrate himself in the one idea that leads from activity to the quiescence of status. The Rajayogic concentration has several stages, that in which the object is seized, that in which it is held, that in which the mind is lost in the status which the object represents or to which the concentration leads, and only the last is termed Samadhi in the Rajayoga although the word is capable, as in the Gita, of a much wider sense. But in the Rajayogic Samadhi there are different grades of status, —that in which the mind, though lost to outward objects, still muses, thinks, perceives in the world of thought, that in which the mind is still capable of primary thought-formations and that in which, all out-darting of the mind even within itself having ceased, the soul rises beyond thought into the silence of the Incommunicable and Ineffable. In all Yoga there are indeed many preparatory objects of thought-concentration, forms, verbal formulas of thought, significant names, all of which are supports[3] to the mind in this movement, all of which have to be used and transcended; the highest support according to the Upanishads is the mystic syllable AUM, whose three letters represent the Brahman or Supreme Self in its three degrees of status, the Waking Soul, the Dream Soul and the Sleep Soul, and the whole potent sound rises towards that which is beyond status as beyond activity.[4]

For of all Yoga of knowledge the final goal is the Transcendent.

We have, however, conceived as the aim of an integral Yoga something more complex and less exclusive—less exclusively positive of the highest condition of the soul, less exclusively negative of its divine radiations. We must aim indeed at the Highest, the Source of all, the Transcendent but not to the exclusion of that which it transcends, rather as the source of an established experience and supreme state of the soul which shall transform all other states and remould our consciousness of the world into the form of its secret Truth. We do not seek to excise from our being all consciousness of the universe, but to realise God, Truth and Self in the universe as well as transcendent of it. We shall seek therefore not only the Ineffable, but also His manifestation as infinite being, consciousness and bliss embracing the universe and at play in it. For that triune infinity is His supreme manifestation and that we shall aspire to know, to share in and to become; and since we seek to realise this Trinity not only in itself but in its cosmic play, we shall aspire also to knowledge of and participation in the universal divine Truth, Knowledge, Will, Love which are His secondary manifestation, His divine becoming. With this too we shall aspire to identify ourselves, towards this too we shall strive to rise and, when the period of effort is passed, allow it by our renunciation of all egoism to draw us up into itself in our being and to descend into us and embrace us in all our becoming. This not only as a means of approach and passage to His supreme transcendence, but as the condition, even when we possess and are possessed by the Transcendent, of a divine life in the manifestation of the cosmos.

In order that we may do this, the terms concentration and Samadhi must assume for us a richer and profound meaning. All our concentration is merely an image of the divine Tapas by which the Self dwells gathered in itself, by which it manifests within itself, by which it maintains and possesses its manifestation, by which it draws back from all manifestation into its supreme oneness. Being dwelling in consciousness upon itself for bliss, this is the divine Tapas; and a Knowledge-Will dwelling in force of consciousness on itself and its manifestations is the essence of the divine concentration, the Yoga of the Lord of Yoga. Given the self-differentiation of the Divine in which we dwell, concentration is the means by which the individual soul identifies itself with and enters into any form, state or psychological self-manifestation (*bhāva*) of the Self. To use this means for unification with the Divine is the condition for the attainment of divine knowledge and the principle of all Yoga of knowledge.

This concentration proceeds by the Idea, using thought, form and name as keys which yield up to the concentrating mind the Truth that lies concealed behind all thought, form and name; for it is through the Idea that the mental being rises beyond all expression to that which is expressed, to that of which the Idea itself is only the instrument. By concentration upon the Idea the mental existence which at present we are breaks open the barrier of our mentality and arrives at the state of consciousness, the state of being, the state of power of conscious-being and bliss of conscious-being to which the Idea corresponds and of which it is the symbol, movement and rhythm. Concentration by the Idea is, then, only a means, a key to open to us the superconscient planes of our existence; a certain self-gathered state of our whole existence lifted into that superconscient truth, unity and infinity of self-aware, self-blissful existence is the aim and culmination; and that is the meaning we shall give to the term Samadhi. Not merely a state withdrawn from all consciousness of the outward, withdrawn even from all consciousness of the inward into that which exists beyond both whether as seed of both or transcendent even of their seed-state; but a settled existence in the One and Infinite, united and identified with it, and this status to remain whether we abide in the waking condition in which we are conscious of the forms of things or we withdraw into the inward activity which dwells in the play of the principles of things, the play of their names and typal forms or we soar to the condition of static inwardness where we arrive at the principles themselves and at the principle of all principles, the seed of name and form.[5]

For the soul that has arrived at the essential Samadhi and is settled in it (*samādhistha*) in the sense the Gita attaches to the word, has that which is fundamental to all experience and cannot fall from it by any experience however distracting to one who has not yet ascended the summit. It can embrace all in the scope of its being without being bound by any or deluded or limited.

When we arrive at this state, all our being and consciousness being concentrated, the necessity of concentration in the Idea ceases. For there in that supramental state the whole position of things is reversed. The mind is a thing that dwells in diffusion, in succession; it can only concentrate on one thing at a time and when not concentrated runs from one thing to another very much at random. Therefore it has to concentrate on a single idea, a single subject of meditation, a single object of contemplation, a single object of will in order to possess or master it, and this it must do to at least the temporary exclusion of all others. But that which is beyond the mind and into which we seek to rise is superior to the running process of the thought, superior to the division of ideas. The Divine is centred in itself and when it throws out ideas and activities does not divide itself or imprison itself in them, but holds them and their movement in its infinity; undivided, its whole self is behind each Idea and each movement and at the same time behind all of them together. Held by it, each spontaneously works itself out, not through a separate act of will, but by the general force of consciousness behind it; if to us there seems to be a concentration of divine Will and Knowledge in each, it is a multiple and equal and not an exclusive concentration, and the reality of it is rather a free and spontaneous working in a self-gathered unity and infinity. The soul which has risen to the divine Samadhi participates in the measure of its attainment in this reversed condition of things,—the true condition, for that which is the reverse of our mentality is the truth. It is for this reason that, as is said in the ancient books, the man who has arrived at Self-possession attains spontaneously without the need of concentration in thought and effort the knowledge or the result which the Idea or the Will in him moves out to embrace.

To arrive then at this settled divine status must be the object of our concentration. The first step in concentration must be always to accustom the discursive mind to a settled unwavering pursuit of a single course of connected thought on a single subject and this it must do undistracted by all lures and alien calls on its attention. Such concentration is common enough in our ordinary life, but it becomes more difficult when we have to do it inwardly without any outward object or action on which to keep the mind; yet this inward concentration is what the seeker of knowledge must effect.[6] Nor must it be merely the consecutive thought of the intellectual thinker, whose only object is to conceive and intellectually link together his conceptions. It is not, except perhaps at first, a process of reasoning that is wanted so much as a dwelling so far as possible on the fruitful essence of the idea which by the insistence of the soul's will upon it must yield up all the facets of its truth. Thus if it be the divine Love that is the subject of concentration, it is on the essence of the idea of God as Love that the mind should concentrate in such a way that the various manifestation of the divine Love should arise luminously, not only to the thought, but in the heart and being and vision of the sadhaka. The thought may come first and the experience afterwards, but equally the experience may come first and the knowledge arise out of the experience. Afterwards the thing attained has to be dwelt on and more and more held till it becomes a constant experience and finally the dharma or law of the being.

This is the process of concentrated meditation; but a more strenuous method is the fixing of the whole mind in concentration on the essence of the idea only, so as to reach not the thought-knowledge or the psychological experience of the subject, but the very essence of the thing behind the idea. In this process thought ceases and passes into the absorbed or ecstatic contemplation of the object or by a merging into it in an inner Samadhi. If this be the process followed, then subsequently the state into which we rise must still be called down to take possession of the lower being, to shed its light, power and bliss on our ordinary consciousness. For otherwise we may possess it, as many do, in the elevated condition or in the inward Samadhi, but we shall lose our hold of it when we awake or descend into the contacts of the world; and this truncated possession is not the aim of an integral Yoga.

A third process is neither at first to concentrate in a strenuous meditation on the one subject nor in a strenuous contemplation of the one object of thought-vision, but first to still the mind altogether. This may be done by various ways; one is to stand back from the mental action altogether not participating in but simply watching it until, tired of its unsanctioned leaping and running, it falls into an increasing and finally an absolute quiet. Another is to reject the thought-suggestions, to cast them away from the mind whenever they come and firmly hold to the peace of the being which really and always exists behind the trouble and riot of the mind. When this secret peace is unveiled, a great calm settles on the being and there comes usually with it the perception and experience of the all-pervading silent Brahman, everything else at first seeming to be mere form and eidolon. On the basis of this calm everything else may be built up in the knowledge and experience no longer of the external phenomena of things but of the deeper truth of the divine manifestation.

Ordinarily, once this state is obtained, strenuous concentration will be found no longer necessary. A free concentration of will[7] using thought merely for suggestion and the giving of light to the lower members will take its place. This Will will then insist on the physical being, the vital existence, the heart and the mind remoulding themselves in the forms of the Divine which reveal themselves out of the silent Brahman. By swifter or slower degrees according to the previous preparation and purification of the members, they will be obliged with more or less struggle to obey the law of the will and its thought-suggestion, so that eventually the knowledge of the Divine takes possession of our consciousness on all its planes and the image of the Divine is formed in our human existence even as it was done by the old Vedic Sadhakas. For the integral Yoga this is the most direct and powerful discipline.

---

1. bāhyasparśa.
2. yato naiva nivartante tad dhāma paramaṁ mama.
3. avalambana.
4. Mandukya Upanishad.

5. The Waking, Dream and Sleep states of the soul.
6. In the elementary stages of internal debate and judgment, *vitarka* and *vicāra*, for the correction of false ideas and arrival at the intellectual truth.
7. This subject will be dealt with more in detail when we come to the Yoga of self-perfection.

# RENUNCIATION

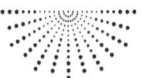

IF DISCIPLINE of all the members of our being by purification and concentration may be described as the right arm of the body of Yoga, renunciation is its left arm. By discipline or positive practice we confirm in ourselves the truth of things, truth of being, truth of knowledge, truth of love, truth of works and replace with these the falsehoods that have overgrown and perverted our nature; by renunciation we seize upon the falsehoods, pluck up their roots and cast them out of our way so that they shall no longer hamper by their persistence, their resistance or their recurrence the happy and harmonious growth of our divine living. Renunciation is an indispensable instrument of our perfection.

How far shall this renunciation go? what shall be its nature? and in what way shall it be applied? There is an established tradition long favoured by great religious teachings and by men of profound spiritual experience that renunciation must not only be complete as a discipline but definite and final as an end and that it shall fall nothing short of the renunciation of life itself and of our mundane existence. Many causes have contributed to the growth of this pure, lofty and august tradition. There is first the profounder cause of the radical opposition between the sullied and imperfect nature of life in the world as it now is in the present stage of our human evolution and the nature of spiritual living; and this opposition has led to the entire rejection of world-existence as a lie, an insanity of the soul, a troubled and unhappy dream or at best a flawed, specious and almost worthless good or to its characterisation as a kingdom of the world, the flesh and the devil, and therefore for the divinely led and divinely attracted soul only a place of ordeal and preparation or at best a play of the All-existence, a game of cross-purposes which He tires of and abandons. A second cause is the soul's hunger for personal salvation, for escape into some farther or farthest height of unalloyed bliss and peace untroubled by the labour and the struggle; or else it is its unwillingness to return from the ecstasy of the divine embrace into the lower field of work and service. But there are other slighter causes incidental to spiritual experience,—strong feeling and practical proof of the great difficulty, which we willingly exaggerate into an impossibility, of combining the life of works and action with spiritual peace and the life of realisation; or else the joy which the mind comes to take in the mere act and state of renunciation,—as it comes indeed to take joy in anything that it has attained or to which it has inured itself,— and the sense of peace and deliverance which is gained by indifference to the world and to the objects of man's desire. Lowest causes of all are the weakness that shrinks from the struggle, the disgust and disappointment of the soul baffled by the great cosmic labour, the selfishness that cares not what becomes of those left behind us so long as we personally can be free from the monstrous ever-circling wheel of death and rebirth, the indifference to the cry that rises up from a labouring humanity.

For the sadhaka of an integral Yoga none of these reasons are valid. With weakness and selfishness, however spiritual in their guise or trend, he can have no dealings; a divine strength and courage and a divine compassion and helpfulness are the very stuff of that which he would be, they are that very nature of the Divine which he would take upon himself as a robe of spiritual light and beauty. The revolvings of the great wheel bring to him no sense of terror or giddiness; he rises above it in his soul and knows from above their divine law and their divine purpose. The difficulty of harmonising the divine life with human living, of being in God and yet living in man is the very difficulty that he is set here to solve and not to shun. He has learned that the joy, the peace and the deliverance are an imperfect crown and no real possession if they do not form a state secure in itself, inalienable to the soul, not dependent on aloofness and inaction but firm in the storm and the race and the battle, unsullied whether by the joy of the world or by its suffering. The ecstasy of the divine embrace will not abandon him because he obeys the impulse of divine love for God in humanity; or if it seems to draw back from him for a while, he knows by experience that it is to try and test him still farther so that some imperfection in his own way of meeting it may fall away from him. Personal salvation he does not seek except as a necessity for the human fulfilment and because he who is himself in bonds cannot easily free others,—though to God nothing is impossible; for a heaven of personal joys he has no hankerings even as a hell of personal sufferings has for him no terrors. If there is an opposition between the spiritual life and that of the world, it is that gulf which he is here to bridge, that opposition which he is here to change into a harmony. If the world is ruled by the flesh and the devil, all the more reason that the children of Immortality should be here to conquer it for God and the Spirit. If life is an insanity, then there are so many million souls to whom there must be brought the light of divine reason; if a dream, yet is it real within itself to so many dreamers who must be brought either to dream nobler dreams or to awaken; or if a lie, then the truth has to be given to the deluded. Nor, if it be said that only by the luminous example of escape from the world can we help the world, shall we accept that dogma, since the contrary example of great Avataras is there to show that not only by rejecting the life of the world as it is can we help, but also and more by accepting and uplifting it. And if it is a play of the All-Existence, then we may well consent to play out our part in it with grace and courage, well take delight in the game along with our divine Playmate.

But, most of all, the view we have taken of the world forbids the renunciation of world-existence so long as we can be anything to God and man in their working-out of its purposes. We regard the world not as an invention of the devil or a self-delusion of the soul, but as a manifestation of the Divine, although as yet a partial because a progressive and evolutionary manifestation. Therefore for us renunciation of life cannot be the goal of life nor rejection of the world the object for which the world was created. We seek to realise our unity with God, but for us that realisation involves a complete and absolute recognition of our unity with man and we cannot cut the two asunder. To use Christian language, the Son of God is also the Son of Man and both elements are necessary to the complete Christhood; or to use an Indian form of thought, the divine Narayana of whom the universe is only one ray is revealed and fulfilled in man; the complete man is Nara-Narayana and in that completeness he symbolises the supreme mystery of existence.

Therefore renunciation must be for us merely an instrument and not an object; nor can it be the only or the chief instrument since our object is the fulfilment of the Divine in the human being, a positive aim which cannot be reached by negative means. The negative means can only be for the removal of that which stands in the way of the positive fulfilment. It must be a renunciation, a complete renunciation of all that is other than and opposed to the divine self-fulfilment and a progressive renunciation of all that is a lesser or only a partial achievement. We shall have no attachment to our life in the world; if that attachment exists, we must renounce it and renounce utterly; but neither shall we have any attachment to the escape from the world, to salvation, to the great self-annihilation; if that attachment exists, that also we must renounce and renounce it utterly.

Again our renunciation must obviously be an inward renunciation; especially and above all, a renunciation of attachment and the craving of desire in the senses and the heart, of self-will in the thought and action and of egoism in the centre of the consciousness. For these things are the three knots by which we are bound to our lower nature and if we can renounce these utterly, there is nothing else that can bind us. Therefore attachment and desire must be utterly cast out; there is nothing in the world to which we must be attached, not wealth nor poverty, nor joy nor suffering, nor life nor death, nor greatness nor littleness, nor vice nor virtue, nor friend, nor wife, nor children, nor country, nor our work and mission, nor heaven nor earth, nor all that is within them or beyond them. And this does not mean that there is nothing at all that we shall love, nothing in which we shall take delight; for attachment is egoism in love and not love itself, desire is limitation and insecurity in a hunger for pleasure and satisfaction and not the seeking after the divine delight in things. A universal love we must have, calm and yet eternally intense beyond the brief vehemence of the most violent passion; a delight in things rooted in a delight in God that does not adhere to their forms but to that which they conceal in themselves and that embraces the universe without being caught in its meshes.[1]

Self-will in thought and action has, we have already seen, to be quite renounced if we would be perfect in the way of divine works; it has equally to be renounced if we are to be perfect in divine knowledge. This self-will means an egoism in the mind which attaches itself to its preferences, its habits, its past or present formations of thought and view and will because it regards them as itself or its own, weaves around them the delicate threads of "I-ness" and "my-ness" and lives in them like a spider in its web. It hates to be disturbed, as a spider hates attack on its web, and feels foreign and unhappy if transplanted to fresh view-points and formations as a spider feels foreign in another web than its own. This attachment must be entirely excised from the mind. Not only must we give up the ordinary attitude to the world and life to which the unawakened mind clings as its natural element; but we must not remain bound in any mental construction of our own or in any intellectual thought-system or arrangement of religious dogmas or logical conclusions; we must not only cut asunder the snare of the mind and the senses, but flee also beyond the snare of the thinker, the snare of the theologian and the hurch-builder, the meshes of the Word and the bondage of the Idea. All these are within us waiting to wall in the spirit with forms; but we must always go beyond, always renounce the lesser for the greater, the finite for the Infinite; we must be prepared to proceed from illumination to illumination, from experience to experience, from soul-state to soul-state so as to reach the utmost transcendence of the Divine and its utmost universality. Nor must we attach ourselves even to the truths we hold most securely, for they are but forms and expressions of the Ineffable who refuses to limit himself to any form or expression; always we must keep ourselves open to the higher Word from above that does not confine itself to its own sense and the light of the Thought that carries in it its own opposites.

But the centre of all resistance is egoism and this we must pursue into every covert and disguise and drag it out and slay it; for its disguises are endless and it will cling to every shred of possible self-concealment. Altruism and indifference are often its most effective disguises; so draped, it will riot boldly in the very face of the divine spies who are missioned to hunt it out. Here the formula of the supreme knowledge comes to our help; we have nothing to do in our essential standpoint with these distinctions, for there is no I nor thou, but only one divine Self equal in all embodiments, equal in the individual and the group, and to realise that, to express that, to serve that, to fulfil that is all that matters. Self-satisfaction and altruism, enjoyment and indifference are not the essential thing. If the realisation, fulfilment, service of the one Self demands from us an action that seems to others self-service or self-assertion in the egoistic sense or seems egoistic enjoyment and self-indulgence, that action we must do; we must be governed by the guide within rather than by the opinions of men. The influence of the environment works often with great subtlety; we prefer and put on almost unconsciously the garb which will look best in the eye that regards us from outside and we allow a veil to drop over the eye within; we are impelled to drape ourselves in the vow of poverty, or in the garb of service, or in outward proofs of indifference and renunciation and a spotless sainthood because that is what tradition and opinion demand of us and so we can make best an impression on our environment. But all this is vanity and delusion. We may be called upon to assume these things, for that may be the uniform of our service; but equally it may not. The eye of man outside matters nothing; the eye within is all.

We see in the teaching of the Gita how subtle a thing is the freedom from egoism which is demanded. Arjuna is driven to fight by the egoism of strength, the egoism of the Kshatriya; he is turned from the battle by the contrary egoism of weakness, the shrinking, the spirit of disgust, the false pity that overcomes the mind, the nervous being and the senses,—not that divine compassion which strengthens the arm and clarifies the knowledge. But this weakness comes garbed as renunciation, as virtue: "Better the life of the beggar than to taste these blood-stained enjoyments; I desire not the rule of all the earth, no, nor the kingdom of the gods." How foolish of the Teacher, we might say, not to confirm this mood, to lose this sublime chance of adding one more great soul to the army of Sannyasins, one more shining example before the world of a holy renunciation. But the Guide sees otherwise, the Guide who is not to be deceived by words; "This is weakness and delusion and egoism that speak in thee. Behold the Self, open thy eyes to the knowledge, purify thy soul of egoism." And afterwards? "Fight, conquer, enjoy a wealthy kingdom." Or to take another example from ancient Indian tradition. It was egoism, it would seem, that drove Rama, the Avatara, to raise an army and destroy a nation in order to recover his wife from the King of Lanka. But would it have been a lesser egoism to drape himself in indifference and misusing the formal terms of the knowledge to say, "I have no wife, no enemy, no desire; these are illusions of the senses; let me cultivate the Brahman-knowledge and let Ravana do what he will with the daughter of Janaka"?

The criterion is within, as the Gita insists. It is to have the soul free from craving and attachment, but free from the attachment to inaction as well as from the egoistic impulse to action, free from attachment to the forms of virtue as well as from the attraction to sin. It is to be rid of "I-ness" and "myness" so as to live in the one Self and act in the one Self; to reject the egoism of refusing to work through the individual centre of the universal Being as well as the egoism of serving the individual mind and life and body to the exclusion of others. To live in the Self is not to dwell for oneself alone in the Infinite immersed and oblivious of all things in that ocean of impersonal self-delight; but it is to live as the Self and in the Self equal in this embodiment and all embodiments and beyond all embodiments. This is the integral knowledge.

It will be seen that the scope we give to the idea of renunciation is different from the meaning currently attached to it. Currently its meaning is self-denial, inhibition of pleasure, rejection of the objects of pleasure. Self-denial is a necessary discipline for the soul of man, because his heart is ignorantly attached; inhibition of pleasure is necessary because his sense is caught and clogged in the mud-honey of sensuous satisfactions; rejection of the objects of pleasure is imposed because the mind fixes on the object and will not leave it to go beyond it and within itself. If the mind of man were not thus ignorant, attached, bound even in its restless inconstancy, deluded by the forms of things, renunciation would not have been needed; the soul could have travelled on the path of delight, from the lesser to the greater, from joy to diviner joy. At present that is not practicable. It must give up from within everything to which it is attached in order that it may gain that which they are in their reality. The external renunciation is not the essential, but even that is necessary for a time, indispensable in many things and sometimes useful in all; we may even say that a complete external renunciation is a stage through which the soul must pass at some period of its progress,— though always it should be without those self-willed violences and fierce self-torturings which are an offence to the Divine seated within us. But in the end this renunciation or self-denial is always an instrument and the period for its use passes. The rejection of the object ceases to be necessary when the object can no longer ensnare us because what the soul enjoys is no longer the object as an object but the Divine which it expresses; the inhibition of pleasure is no longer needed when the soul no longer seeks pleasure but possesses the delight of the Divine in all things equally without the need of a personal or physical possession of the thing itself; self-denial loses its field when the soul no longer claims anything, but obeys consciously the will of the one Self in all beings. It is then that we are freed from the Law and released into the liberty of the Spirit.

We must be prepared to leave behind on the path not only that which we stigmatise as evil, but that which seems to us to be good, yet is not the one good. There are things which were beneficial, helpful, which seemed perhaps at one time the one thing desirable, and yet once their work is done, once they are attained, they become obstacles and even hostile forces when we are called to advance beyond them. There are desirable states of the soul which it is dangerous to rest in after they have been mastered, because then we do not march on to the wider kingdoms of God beyond. Even divine realisations must not be clung to, if they are not the divine realisation in its utter essentiality and completeness. We must rest at nothing less than the All, nothing short of the utter transcendence. And if we can thus be free in the spirit, we shall find out all the wonder of God's workings; we shall find that in inwardly renouncing everything we have lost nothing. "By all this abandoned thou shalt come to enjoy the All." For everything is kept for us and restored to us but with a wonderful change and transfiguration into the All-Good and the All-Beautiful, the All-Light and the All-Delight of Him who is for ever pure and infinite and the mystery and the miracle that ceases not through the ages.

---

1. *Nirlipta.* The divine Ananda in things is *niṣkāma* and *nirlipta,* free from desire and therefore not attached.

# THE SYNTHESIS OF THE DISCIPLINES
## OF KNOWLEDGE

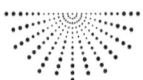

IN THE last chapter we have spoken of renunciation in its most general scope, even as we spoke of concentration in all its possibilities; what has been said, applies therefore equally to the path of Works and the path of Devotion as to the path of Knowledge; for on all three concentration and renunciation are needed, though the way and spirit in which they are applied may vary. But we must now turn more particularly to the actual steps of the Path of Knowledge on which the double force of concentration and renunciation must aid us to advance. Practically, this path is a reascent up the great ladder of being down which the soul has descended into the material existence.

The central aim of Knowledge is the recovery of the Self, of our true self-existence, and this aim presupposes the admission that our present mode of being is not our true self-existence. No doubt, we have rejected the trenchant solutions which cut the knot of the riddle of the universe; we recognise it neither as a fiction of material appearance created by Force, nor as an unreality set up by the Mind, nor as a bundle of sensations, ideas and results of idea and sensation with a great Void or a great blissful Zero behind it to strive towards as our true truth of eternal non-existence. We accept the Self as a reality and the universe as a reality of the Self, a reality of its consciousness and not of mere material force and formation, but none the less or rather all the more for that reason a reality. Still, though the universe is a fact and not a fiction, a fact of the divine and universal and not a fiction of the individual self, our state of existence here is a state of ignorance, not the true truth of our being. We conceive of ourselves falsely, we see ourselves as we are not; we live in a false relation with our environment, because we know neither the universe nor ourselves for what they really are but with an imperfect view founded on a temporary fiction which the Soul and Nature have established between themselves for the convenience of the evolving ego. And this falsity is the root of a general perversion, confusion and suffering which besiege at every step both our internal life and our relations with our environment. Our personal life and our communal life, our commerce with ourselves and our commerce with our fellows are founded on a falsity and are therefore false in their recognised principles and methods, although through all this error a growing truth continually seeks to express itself. Hence the supreme importance to man of Knowledge, not what is called the practical knowledge of life, but of the profoundest knowledge of the Self and Nature[1] on which alone a true practice of life can be founded.

The error proceeds from a false identification. Nature has created within her material unity separate-seeming bodies which the Soul manifested in material Nature enfolds, inhabits, possesses, uses; the Soul forgetting itself experiences only this single knot in Matter and says "I am this body." It thinks of itself as the body, suffers with the body, enjoys with the body, is born with the body, is dissolved with the body; or so at least it views its self-existence. Again, Nature has created within her unity of universal life separate-seeming currents of life which form themselves into a whorl of vitality around and in each body, and the Soul manifested in vital Nature seizes on and is seized by that current, is imprisoned momentarily in that little whirling vortex of live. The Soul, still forgetting itself, says "I am this life"; it thinks of itself as the life, craves with its cravings or desires, wallows in its pleasures, bleeds with its wounds, rushes or stumbles with its movements. If it is still mainly governed by the body-sense, it identifies its own existence with that of the whorl and thinks "When this whorl is dissipated by the dissolution of the body round which it has formed itself, then *I* shall be no more." If it has been able to sense the current of life which has formed the vortex, it thinks of itself as that current and says "I am this stream of life; I have entered upon the possession of this body, I shall leave it and enter upon the possession of other bodies: I am an immortal life revolving in a cycle of constant rebirth."

But again Nature has created within her mental unity, formed in the universal Mind separate-seeming dynamos as it were of mentality, constant centres for the generation, distribution and reabsorption of mental force and mental activities, stations as it were in a system of mental telegraphy where messages are conceived, written, sent, received, deciphered, and these messages and these activities are of many kinds, sensational, emotional, perceptual, conceptual, intuitional, all of which the Soul manifested in mental Nature accepts, uses for its outlook on the world and seems to itself to project and to receive their shocks, to suffer or to master their consequences. Nature instals the base of these dynamos in the material bodies she has formed, makes these bodies the ground for her stations and connects the mental with the material by a nerve-system full of the movement of vital currents through which the mind becomes conscious of the material world and, so far as it chooses, of the vital world of Nature. Otherwise the mind would be conscious of the mental world first and chiefly and would only indirectly glimpse the material. As it is, its attention is fixed on the body and the material world in which it has been installed and it is aware of the rest of existence only dimly, indirectly or subconsciously in that vast remainder of itself with regard to which superficially it has become irresponsive and oblivious.

The Soul identifies itself with this mental dynamo or station and says "I am this mind." And since the mind is absorbed in the bodily life, it thinks "I am a mind in a living body" or, still more commonly, "I am a body which lives and thinks." It identifies itself with the thoughts, emotions, sensations of the embodied mind and imagines that because when the body is dissolved all this will dissolve, itself also will cease to exist. Or if it becomes conscious of the current of persistence of mental personality, it thinks of itself as a mental soul occupying the body whether once or repeatedly and returning from earthly living to mental worlds beyond; the persistence of this mental being mentally enjoying or suffering sometimes in the body, sometimes on the mental or vital plane of Nature it calls its immortal existence. Or else, because the mind is a principle of light and knowledge, however imperfect, and can have some notion of what is beyond it, it sees the possibility of a dissolution of the mental being into that which is beyond, some Void or some eternal Existence, and it says, "There I, the mental soul, cease to be." Such dissolution it dreads or desires, denies or affirms according to its measure of attachment to or repulsion from this present play of embodied mind and vitality.

Now, all this is a mixture of truth and falsehood. Mind, Life, Matter exist and mental, vital, physical individualisation exists as facts in Nature, but the identification of the soul with these things is a false identification. Mind, Life and Matter are ourselves only in this sense that they are principles of being which the true self has evolved by the meeting and interaction of Soul and Nature in order to express a form of its one existence as the Cosmos. Individual mind, life and body are a play of these principles which is set up in the commerce of Soul and Nature as a means for the expression of that multiplicity of itself of which the one Existence is eternally capable and which it holds eternally involved in its unity. Individual mind, life and body are forms of ourselves in so far as we are centres of the multiplicity of the One; universal Mind, Life and Body are also forms of our self, because we are that One in our being. But the self is more than universal or individual mind, life and body and when we limit ourselves by identification with these things, we found our knowledge on a falsehood, we falsify our determining view and our practical experience not only of our self-being but of our cosmic existence and of our individual activities.

The Self is an eternal utter Being and pure existence of which all these things are becomings. From this knowledge we have to proceed; this knowledge we have to realise and make it the foundation of the inner and the outer life of the individual. The Yoga of Knowledge, starting from this primary truth, has conceived a negative and positive method of discipline by which we shall get rid of these false identifications and recoil back from them into true self-knowledge. The negative method is to say always "I am not the body" so as to contradict and root out the false idea "I am the body", to concentrate on this knowledge and by renunciation of the attachment of the soul to the physical get rid of the body-sense. We say again "I am not the life" and by concentration on this knowledge and renunciation of attachment to the vital movements and desires, get rid of the life-sense. We say, finally, "I am not the mind, the motion, the sense, the thought" and by concentration on this knowledge and renunciation of the mental activities, get rid of the mind-sense. When we thus constantly create a gulf between ourselves and the things with which we identified ourselves, their veils progressively fall away from us and the Self begins to be visible to our experience. Of that then we say "I am That, the pure, the eternal, the self-blissful" and by concentrating our thought and being upon it we become That and are able finally to renounce the individual existence and the Cosmos. Another positive method belonging rather to the Rajayoga is to concentrate on the thought of the Brahman and shut out from us all other ideas, so that this dynamo of mind shall cease to work upon our external or varied internal existence; by mental cessation the vital and physical play also shall fall to rest in an eternal samadhi, some inexpressible deepest trance of the being in which we shall pass into the absolute Existence.

This discipline is evidently a self-centred and exclusive inner movement which gets rid of the world by denying it in thought and shutting the eyes of the soul to it in vision. But the universe is there as a truth in God even though the individual soul may have shut its eyes to it and the Self is there in the universe really and not falsely, supporting all that we have rejected, truly immanent in all things, really embracing the individual in the universal as well as embracing the universe in that which exceeds and transcends it. What shall we do with this eternal Self in this persistent universe which we see encompassing us every time we come out of the trance of inner meditation? The ascetic Path of Knowledge has its solution and its discipline for the soul that looks out on the universe. It is to regard the immanent and all-encompassing and all-constituting Self in the image of the ether in which all forms are, which is in all forms, of which all forms are made. In that ether cosmic Life and Mind move as the Breath of things, an atmospheric sea in the ethereal, and constitute from it all these forms; but what they constitute are merely name and form and not realities; the form of the pot we see is a form of earth only and goes back into the earth, earth a form resolvable into the cosmic Life, the cosmic Life a movement that falls to rest in that silent immutable Ether. Concentrating on this knowledge, rejecting all phenomenon and appearance, we come to see the whole as an illusion of name and form in the ether that is Brahman; it becomes unreal to us; and the universe becoming unreal the immanence becomes unreal and there is only the Self upon which our mind has falsely imposed the name and form of the universe. Thus are we justified in the withdrawal of the individual self into the Absolute.

Still, the Self goes on with its imperishable aspect of immanence, its immutable aspect of divine envelopment, its endless trick of becoming each thing and all things; our detection of the cheat and our withdrawal do not seem to affect one tittle either the Self or the universe. Must we not then know also what it is that thus persists superior to our acceptance and rejection and too great, too eternal to be affected by it? Here too there must be some invincible reality at work and the integrality of

Knowledge demands that we shall see and realise it; otherwise it may prove that our own knowledge and not the Lord in the universe was the cheat and the illusion. Therefore we must concentrate again and see and realise also this which persists so sovereignly and must know the Self as no other than the Supreme Soul which is the Lord of Nature, the upholder of cosmic existence by whose sanction it proceeds, whose will compels its multitudinous actions and determines its perpetual cycles. And we must yet concentrate once again and see and realise and must know the Self as the one Existence who is both the Soul of all and the Nature of all, at once Purusha and Prakriti and so able both to express himself in all these forms of things and to be all these formations. Otherwise we have excluded what the Self does not exclude and made a wilful choice in our knowledge.

The old ascetic Path of Knowledge admitted the unity of things and the concentration on all these aspects of the one Existence, but it made a distinction and a hierarchy. The Self that becomes all these forms of things is the Virat or universal Soul; the Self that creates all these forms is Hiranyagarbha, the luminous or creatively perceptive Soul; the Self that contains all these things involved in it is Prajna, the conscious Cause or originally determining Soul; beyond all these is the Absolute who permits all this unreality, but has no dealings with it. Into That we must withdraw and have no farther dealings with the universe, since Knowledge means the final Knowledge, and therefore these lesser realisations must fall away from us or be lost in That. But evidently from our point of view these are practical distinctions made by the mind which have a value for certain purposes, but no ultimate value. Our view of the world insists on unity; the universal Self is not different from the perceptive and creative, nor the perceptive from the causal, nor the causal from the Absolute, but it is one "Self-being which has become all becomings", and which is not any other than the Lord who manifests Himself as all these individual existences nor the Lord any other than the sole-existing Brahman who verily is all this that we can see, sense, live or mentalise. That Self, Lord, Brahman we would know that we may realise our unity with it and with all that it manifests and in that unity we would live. For we demand of knowledge that it shall unite; the knowledge that divides must always be a partial knowing good for certain practical purposes; the knowledge that unites is *the* knowledge.

Therefore our integral Yoga will take up these various disciplines and concentrations, but harmonise and if possible fuse them by a synthesis which removes their mutual exclusions. Not realising the Lord and the All only to reject them for silent Self or unknowable Absolute as would an exclusively transcendental, nor living for the Lord alone or in the All alone as would an exclusively theistic or an exclusively pantheistic Yoga, the seeker of integral knowledge will limit himself neither in his thought nor in his practice nor in his realisation by any religious creed or philosophical dogma. He will seek the Truth of existence in its completeness. The ancient disciplines he will not reject, for they rest upon eternal truths, but he will give them an orientation in conformity with his aim.

We must recognise that our primary aim in knowledge must be to realise our own supreme Self more than that Self in others or as the Lord of Nature or as the All; for that is the pressing need of the individual, to arrive at the highest truth of his own being, to set right its disorders, confusions, false identifications, to arrive at its right concentration and purity and to know and mount to its source. But we do this not in order to disappear into its source, but so that our whole existence and all the members of this inner kingdom may find their right basis, may live in our highest self, live for our highest self only and obey no other law than that which proceeds from our highest self and is given to our purified being without any falsification in the transmitting mentality. And if we do this rightly we shall discover that in finding this supreme Self we have found the one Self in all, the one Lord of our nature and of all Nature, the All of ourselves who is the All of the universe. For this that we see in ourselves we must necessarily see everywhere, since that in the truth of His unity. By discovering and using rightly the Truth of our being the barrier between our individuality and the universe will necessarily be forced open and cast away and the Truth that we realise in our own being cannot fail to realise itself to us in the universality which will then be our self. Realising in ourselves the "I am He" of the Vedanta, we cannot but realise in looking upon all around us the identical knowledge on its other side, "Thou art That." We have only to see how practically the discipline must be conducted in order that we may arrive successfully at this great unification.

---

1. *ātmajñāna* and *tattvajñāna*.

# THE RELEASE FROM SUBJECTION TO THE BODY

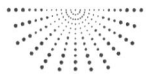

OUR FIRST step in this path of knowledge, having once determined in our intellect that what seems is not the Truth, that the self is not the body or life or mind, since these are only its forms, must be to set right our mind in its practical relation with the life and the body so that it may arrive at its own right relation with the Self. This it is easiest to do by a device with which we are already familiar, since it played a great part in our view of the Yoga of Works; it is to create a separation between the Prakriti and the Purusha. The Purusha, the soul that knows and commands has got himself involved in the workings of his executive conscious force, so that he mistakes this physical working of it which we call the body for himself; he forgets his own nature as the soul that knows and commands; he believes his mind and soul to be subject to the law and working of the body; he forgets that he is so much else besides that is greater than the physical form; he forgets that the mind is really greater than Matter and ought not to submit to its obscurations, reactions, habit of inertia, habit of incapacity; he forgets that he is more even than the mind, a Power which can raise the mental being above itself; that he is the Master, the Transcendent and it is not fit the Master should be enslaved to his own workings, the Transcendent imprisoned in a form which exists only as a trifle in its own being. All this forgetfulness has to be cured by the Purusha remembering his own true nature and first by his remembering that the body is only a working and only one working of Prakriti.

We say then to the mind "This is a working of Prakriti, this is neither thyself nor myself; stand back from it." We shall find, if we try, that the mind has this power of detachment and can stand back from the body not only in idea, but in act and as it were physically or rather vitally. This detachment of the mind must be strengthened by a certain attitude of indifference to the things of the body; we must not care essentially about its sleep or its waking, its movement or its rest, its pain or its pleasure, its health or ill-health, its vigour or its fatigue, its comfort or its discomfort, or what it eats or drinks. This does not mean that we shall not keep the body in right order so far as we can; we have not to fall into violent asceticisms or a positive neglect of the physical frame. But we have not either to be affected in mind by hunger or thirst or discomfort or ill-health or attach the importance which the physical and vital man attaches to the things of the body, or indeed any but a quite subordinate and purely instrumental importance. Nor must this instrumental importance be allowed to assume the proportions of a necessity; we must not for instance imagine that the purity of the mind depends on the things we eat or drink, although during a certain stage restrictions in eating and drinking are useful to our inner progress; nor on the other hand must we continue to think that the dependence of the mind or even of the life on food and drink is anything more than a habit, a customary relation which Nature has set up between these principles. As a matter of fact the food we take can be reduced by contrary habit and new relation to a minimum without the mental or vital vigour being in any way reduced; even on the contrary with a judicious development they can be trained to a greater potentiality of vigour by learning to rely on the secret fountains of mental and vital energy with which they are connected more than upon the minor aid of physical aliments. This aspect of self-discipline is however more important in the Yoga of self-perfection than here; for our present purpose the important point is the renunciation by the mind of attachment to or dependence on the things of the body.

Thus disciplined the mind will gradually learn to take up towards the body the true attitude of the Purusha. First of all, it will know the mental Purusha as the upholder of the body and not in any way the body itself; for it is quite other than the physical existence which it upholds by the mind through the agency of the vital force. This will come to be so much the normal attitude of the whole being to the physical frame that the latter will feel to us as if something external and detachable like the dress we wear or an instrument we happen to be carrying in our hand. We may even come to feel that the body is in a certain sense non-existent except as a sort of partial expression of our vital force and of our mentality. These experiences are signs that the mind is coming to a right poise regarding the body, that it is exchanging the false view-point of the mentality obsessed and captured by physical sensation for the viewpoint of the true truth of things.

Secondly, with regard to the movements and experiences of the body the mind will come to know the Purusha seated within it as, first, the witness or observer of the movements and, secondly, the knower or perceiver of the experiences. It will cease to consider in thought or feel in sensation these movements and experiences as its own but rather consider and feel them as not its own, as operations of Nature governed by the qualities of Nature and their interaction upon each other. This detachment can be made so normal and carried so far that there will be a kind of division between the mind and the body and the former will observe and experience the hunger, thirst, pain, fatigue, depression, etc. of the physical being as if they were experiences of some other person with whom it has so close a *rapport* as to be aware of all that is going on within him. This division is a great means, a great step towards mastery; for the mind comes to observe these things first without being overpowered and finally without being at all affected by them, dispassionately, with clear understanding but with perfect detachment. This is the initial liberation of the mental being from servitude to the body; for by right knowledge put steadily into practice liberation comes inevitably.

Finally, the mind will come to know the Purusha in the mind as the master of Nature whose sanction is necessary to her movements. It will find that as the giver of the sanction he can withdraw the original fiat from the previous habits of Nature and that eventually the habit will cease or change in the direction indicated by the will of the Purusha; not at once, for the old sanction persists as an obstinate consequence of the past Karma of Nature until that is exhausted, and a good deal also depends on the force of the habit and the idea of fundamental necessity which the mind had previously attached to it; but if it is not one of the fundamental habits Nature has established for the relation of the mind, life and body and if the old sanction is not renewed by the mind or the habit willingly indulged, then eventually the change will come. Even the habit of hunger and thirst can be minimised, inhibited, put away; the habit of disease can be similarly minimised and gradually eliminated and in the meantime the power of the mind to set right the disorders of the body whether by conscious manipulation of vital force or by simple mental fiat will immensely increase. By a similar process the habit by which the bodily nature associates certain forms and degrees of activity with strain, fatigue, incapacity can be rectified and the power, freedom, swiftness, effectiveness of the work whether physical or mental which can be done with this bodily instrument marvellously increased, doubled, tripled, decupled.

This side of the method belongs properly to the Yoga of self-perfection; but it is as well to speak briefly of these things here both because we thereby lay a basis for what we shall have to say of self-perfection, which is a part of the integral Yoga, and because we have to correct the false notions popularised by materialistic Science. According to this Science the normal mental and physical states and the relations between mind and body actually established by our past evolution are the right, natural and healthy conditions and anything other, anything opposite to them is either morbid and wrong or a hallucination, self-deception and insanity. Needless to say, this conservative principle is entirely ignored by Science itself when it so diligently and successfully improves on the normal operations of physical Nature for the greater mastery of Nature by man. Suffice it to say here once for all that a change of mental and physical state and of relations between the mind and body which increases the purity and freedom of the being, brings a clear joy and peace and multiplies the power of the mind over itself and over the physical functions, brings about in a word man's greater mastery of his own nature, is obviously not morbid and cannot be considered a hallucination or self-deception since its effects are patent and positive. In fact, it is simply a willed advance of Nature in her evolution of the individual, an evolution which she will carry out in any case but in which she chooses to utilise the human will as her chief agent, because her essential aim is to lead the Purusha to conscious mastery over herself.

This being said, we must add that in the movement of the path of knowledge perfection of the mind and body are no consideration at all or only secondary considerations. The one thing necessary is to rise out of Nature to the Self by either the most swift or the most thorough and effective method possible; and the method we are describing, though not the swiftest, is the most thorough-going in its effectivity. And here there arises the question of physical action or inaction. It is ordinarily considered that the Yogin should draw away from action as much as possible and especially that too much action is a hindrance because it draws off the energies outward. To a certain extent this is true; and we must note farther that when the mental Purusha takes up the attitude of mere witness and observer, a tendency to silence, solitude, physical calm and bodily inaction grows upon the being. So long as this is not associated with inertia, incapacity or unwillingness to act, in a word, with the growth of the tamasic quality, all this is to the good. The power to do nothing, which is quite different from indolence, incapacity or aversion to action and attachment to inaction, is a great power and a great mastery; the power to rest absolutely from action is as necessary for the Jnanayogin as the power to cease absolutely from thought, as the power to remain indefinitely in sheer solitude and silence and as the power of immovable calm. Whoever is not willing to embrace these states is not yet fit for the path that leads towards the highest knowledge; whoever is unable to draw towards them, is as yet unfit for its acquisition.

At the same time it must be added that the power is enough; the abstention from all physical action is not indispensable, the aversion to action mental or corporeal is not desirable. The seeker of the integral state of knowledge must be free from attachment to action and equally free from attachment to inaction. Especially must any tendency to mere inertia of mind or vitality or body be surmounted, and if that habit is found growing on the nature, the will of the Purusha must be used to dismiss it. Eventually, a state arrives when the life and the body perform as mere instruments the will of the Purusha in the mind without any strain or attachment, without their putting themselves into the action with that inferior, eager and often feverish energy which is the nature of their ordinary working; they come to work as forces of Nature work without the fret and toil and reaction characteristic of life in the body when it is not yet master of the physical. When we attain to this perfection, then action and inaction become immaterial, since neither interferes with the freedom of the soul or draws it away from its urge towards the Self or its poise in the Self. But this state of perfection arrives later in the Yoga and till then the law of moderation laid down by the Gita is the best for us; too much mental or physical action then is not good since excess draws away too much energy and reacts unfavourably upon the spiritual condition; too little also is not good since defect leads to a habit of inaction and even to an incapacity which has afterwards to be surmounted with difficulty. Still, periods of absolute calm, solitude and cessation from works are highly desirable and should be secured as often as possible for that recession of the soul into itself which is indispensable to knowledge.

While dealing thus with the body we have necessarily to deal also with the Prana or life-energy. For practical purposes we have to make a distinction between the life-energy as it acts in the body, the physical Prana, and the life-energy as it acts in support of the mental activities, the psychical Prana. For we lead always a double life, mental and physical, and the same life-energy acts differently and assumes a different aspect according as it lends itself to one or the other. In the body it produces those reactions of hunger, thirst, fatigue, health, disease, physical vigour, etc. which are the vital experiences of the physical frame. For the gross body of man is not like the stone or the earth; it is a combination of two sheaths, the vital and the "food" sheath and its life is a constant interaction of these two. Still the life-energy and the physical frame are two different things and in the withdrawal of the mind from the absorbing sense of the body we become increasingly sensible of the Prana and its action in the corporeal instrument and can observe and more and more control its operations. Practically, in drawing back from the body we draw back from the physical life-energy also, even while we distinguish the two and feel the latter nearer to us than the mere physical instrument. The entire conquest of the body comes in fact by the conquest of the physical life-energy.

Along with the attachment to the body and its works the attachment to life in the body is overcome. For when we feel the physical being to be not ourselves, but only a dress or an instrument, the repulsion to the death of the body which is so strong and vehement an instinct of the vital man must necessarily weaken and can be thrown away. Thrown away it must be and entirely. The fear of death and the aversion to bodily cessation are the stigma left by his animal origin on the human being. That brand must be utterly effaced.

# THE RELEASE FROM THE HEART AND THE MIND

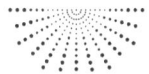

BUT THE ascending soul has to separate itself not only from the life in the body but from the action of the life-energy in the mind; it has to make the mind say as the representative of the Purusha "I am not the Life; the Life is not the self of the Purusha, it is only a working and only one working of Prakriti." The characteristics of Life are action and movement, a reaching out to absorb and assimilate what is external to the individual and a principle of satisfaction or dissatisfaction in what it seizes upon or what comes to it, which is associated with the all-pervading phenomenon of attraction and repulsion. These three things are everywhere in Nature because Life is everywhere in Nature. But in us mental beings they are all given a mental value according to the mind which perceives and accepts them. They take the form of action, of desire and of liking and disliking, pleasure and pain. The Prana is everywhere in us supporting not only the action of our body, but of our sense-mind, our emotional mind, our thought-mind; and bringing its own law or dharma into all these, it confuses, it limits, it throws into discord their right action and creates that impurity of misplacement and that tangled confusion which is the whole evil of our psychological existence. In that confusion one law seems to reign, the law of desire. As the universal Divine Being, all-embracing and all-possessing, acts, moves, enjoys purely for the satisfaction of divine Delight, so the individual life acts, moves, enjoys and suffers predominantly for the satisfaction of desire. Therefore the psychic life-energy presents itself to our experience as a sort of desire-mind, which we have to conquer if we mean to get back to our true self.

Desire is at once the motive of our actions, our lever of accomplishment and the bane of our existence. If our sense-mind, emotional mind, thought-mind could act free from the intrusions and importations of the life-energy, if that energy could be made to obey their right action instead of imposing its own yoke on our existence, all human problems would move harmoniously to their right solution. The proper function of the life-energy is to do what it is bidden by the divine principle in us, to reach to and enjoy what is given to it by that indwelling Divine and not to desire at all. The proper function of the sense-mind is to lie open passively, luminously to the contacts of Life and transmit their sensations and the *rasa* or right taste and principle of delight in them to the higher function; but interfered with by the attractions and repulsions, the acceptances and refusals, the satisfactions and dissatisfactions, the capacities and incapacities of the life-energy in the body it is, to begin with, limited in its scope and, secondly, forced in these limits to associate itself with all these discords of the life in Matter. It becomes an instrument for pleasure and pain instead of for delight of existence.

Similarly the emotional mind compelled to take note of all these discords and subject itself to their emotional reactions becomes a hurtling field of joy and grief, love and hatred, wrath, fear, struggle, aspiration, disgust, likes, dislikes, indifferences, content, discontent, hopes, disappointments, gratitude, revenge and all the stupendous play of passion which is the drama of life in the world. This chaos we call our soul. But the real soul, the real psychic entity which for the most part we see little of and only a small minority in mankind has developed, is an instrument of pure love, joy and the luminous reaching out to fusion and unity with God and our fellow-creatures. This psychic entity is covered up by the play of the mentalised Prana or desire-mind which we mistake for the soul; the emotional mind is unable to mirror the real soul in us, the Divine in our hearts, and is obliged instead to mirror the desire-mind.

So too the proper function of the thought-mind is to observe, understand, judge with a dispassionate delight in knowledge and open itself to messages and illuminations playing upon all that it observes and upon all that is yet hidden from it but must progressively be revealed, messages and illuminations that secretly flash down to us from the divine Oracle concealed in light above our mentality whether they seem to descend through the intuitive mind or arise from the seeing heart. But this it cannot do rightly because it is pinned to the limitations of the life-energy in the senses, to the discords of sensation and emotion, and to its own limitations of intellectual preference, inertia, straining, self-will which are the form taken in it by the interference of this desire-mind, this psychic Prana. As is said in the Upanishads, our whole mind-consciousness is shot through with the threads and currents of this Prana, this Life-energy that strives and limits, grasps and misses, desires and suffers, and only by its purification can we know and possess our real and eternal self.

It is true that the root of all this evil is the ego-sense and that the seat of the conscious ego-sense is the mind itself; but in reality the conscious mind only reflects an ego already created in the subconscious mind in things, the dumb soul in the stone and the plant which is present in all body and life and only finally delivered into voicefulness and wakefulness but not originally created by the conscious mind. And in this upward procession it is the life-energy which has become the obstinate knot of the ego, it is the desire-mind which refuses to relax the knot even when the intellect and the heart have discovered the cause of their ills and would be glad enough to remove it; for the Prana in them is the Animal who revolts and who obscures and deceives their knowledge and coerces their will by his refusal.

Therefore the mental Purusha has to separate himself from association and self-identification with this desire-mind. He has to say "I am not this thing that struggles and suffers, grieves and rejoices, loves and hates, hopes and is baffled, is angry and afraid and cheerful and depressed, a thing of vital moods and emotional passions. All these are merely workings and habits of Prakriti in the sensational and emotional mind." The mind then draws back from its emotions and becomes with these, as with the bodily movements and experiences, the observer or witness. There is again an inner cleavage. There is this emotional mind in which these moods and passions continue to occur according to the habit of the modes of Nature and there is the observing mind which sees them, studies and understands but is detached from them. It observes them as if in a sort of action and play on a mental stage of personages other than itself, at first with interest and a habit of relapse into identification, then with entire calm and detachment, and, finally, attaining not only to calm but to the pure delight of its own silent existence, with a smile at their unreality as at the imaginary joys and sorrows of a child who is playing and loses himself in the play. Secondly, it becomes aware of itself as master of the sanction who by his withdrawal of sanction can make this play to cease. When the sanction is withdrawn, another significant phenomenon takes place; the emotional mind becomes normally calm and pure and free from these reactions, and even when they come, they no longer rise from within but seem to fall on it as impressions from outside to which its fibres are still able to respond; but this habit of response dies away and the emotional mind is in time entirely liberated from the passions which it has renounced. Hope and fear, joy and grief, liking and disliking, attraction and repulsion, content and discontent, gladness and depression, horror and wrath and fear and disgust and shame and the passions of love and hatred fall away from the liberated psychic being.

What takes their place? It may be, if we will, an entire calm, silence and indifference. But although this is a stage through which the soul has usually to pass, it is not the final aim we have placed before us. Therefore the Purusha becomes also the master who wills and whose will it is to replace wrong by right enjoyment of the psychic existence. What he wills, Nature executes. What was fabric-stuff of desire and passion, is turned into reality of pure, equal and calmly intense love and joy and oneness. The real soul emerges and takes the place left vacant by the desire-mind. The cleansed and emptied cup is filled with the wine of divine love and delight and no longer with the sweet and bitter poison of passion. The passions, even the passion for good, misrepresent the divine nature. The passion of pity with its impure elements of physical repulsion and emotional inability to bear the suffering of others has to be rejected and replaced by the higher divine compassion which sees, understands, accepts the burden of others and is strong to help and heal, not with self-will and revolt against the suffering in the world and with ignorant accusation of the law of things and their source, but with light and knowledge and as an instrument of the Divine in its emergence. So too the love that desires and grasps and is troubled with joy and shaken with grief must be rejected for the equal, all-embracing love that is free from these things and has no dependence upon circumstances and is not modified by response or absence of response. So we shall deal with all the movements of the soul; but of these things we shall speak farther when we consider the Yoga of self-perfection.

As with action and inaction, so it is with this dual possibility of indifference and calm on the one side and active joy and love on the other. Equality, not indifference is the basis. Equal endurance, impartial indifference, calm submission to the causes of joy and grief without any reaction of either grief or joy are the preparation and negative basis of equality; but equality is not fulfilled till it takes its positive form of love and delight. The sense-mind must find the equal *rasa* of the All-Beautiful, the heart the equal love and Ananda for all, the psychic Prana the enjoyment of this *rasa*, love and Ananda. This, however, is the positive perfection that comes by liberation; our first object on the path of knowledge is rather the liberation that comes by detachment from the desire-mind and by the renunciation of its passions.

The desire-mind must also be rejected from the instrument of thought and this is best done by the detachment of the Purusha from thought and opinion itself. Of this we have already had occasion to speak when we considered in what consists the integral purification of the being. For all this movement of knowledge which we are describing is a method of purification and liberation whereby entire and final self-knowledge becomes possible, a progressive self-knowledge being itself the instrument of the purification and liberation. The method with the thought-mind will be the same as with all the rest of the being. The Purusha, having used the thought-mind for release from identification with the life and body and with the mind of desire and sensations and emotions, will turn round upon the thought-mind itself and will say "This too I am not; I am not the thought or the thinker; all these ideas, opinions, speculations, strivings of the intellect, its predilections, preferences, dogmas, doubts, self-corrections are not myself; all this is only a working of Prakriti which takes place in the thought-mind." Thus a division is created between the mind that thinks and wills and the mind that observes and the Purusha becomes the witness only; he sees, he understands the process and laws of his thought, but detaches himself from it. Then as the master of the sanction he withdraws his past sanction from the tangle of the mental undercurrent and the reasoning intellect and causes both to cease from their importunities. He becomes liberated from subjection to the thinking mind and capable of the utter silence.

For perfection there is necessary also the resumption by the Purusha of his position as the lord of his Nature and the will to replace the mere mental undercurrent and intellect by the truth-conscious thought that lightens from above. But the silence is necessary; in the silence and not in the thought we shall find the Self, we shall become aware of it, not merely conceive it, and we shall withdraw out of the mental Purusha into that which is the source of the mind. But for this withdrawal a final liberation is needed, the release from the ego-sense in the mind.

# THE RELEASE FROM THE EGO

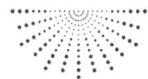

THE FORMATION of a mental and vital ego tied to the body-sense was the first great labour of the cosmic Life in its progressive evolution; for this was the means it found for creating out of matter a conscious individual. The dissolution of this limiting ego is the one condition, the necessary means for this very same Life to arrive at its divine fruition: for only so can the conscious individual find either his transcendent self or his true Person. This double movement is usually represented as a fall and a redemption or a creation and a destruction,—the kindling of a light and its extinction or the formation first of a smaller temporary and unreal self and a release from it into our true self's eternal largeness. For human thought falls apart towards two opposite extremes: one, mundane and pragmatic, regards the fulfilment and satisfaction of the mental, vital and physical ego-sense individual or collective as the object of life and looks no farther, while the other, spiritual, philosophic or religious, regards the conquest of the ego in the interests of the soul, spirit or whatever be the ultimate entity, as the one thing supremely worth doing. Even in the camp of the ego there are two divergent attitudes which divide the mundane or materialist theory of the universe. One tendency of this thought regards the mental ego as a creation of our mentality which will be dissolved with the dissolution of mind by the death of the body; the one abiding truth is eternal Nature working in the race—this or another—and her purpose should be followed, not ours,—

the fulfilment of the race, the collective ego, and not that of the individual should be the rule of life. Another trend of thought, more vitalistic in its tendencies, fixes on the conscious ego as the supreme achievement of Nature, no matter how transitory, ennobles it into a human representative of the Will-to-be and holds up its greatness and satisfaction as the highest aim of our existence. In the more numerous systems that take their stand on some kind of religious thought or spiritual discipline there is a corresponding divergence. The Buddhist denies the existence of a real self or ego, admits no universal or transcendent Being. The Adwaitin declares the apparently individual soul to be none other than the supreme Self and Brahman, its individuality an illusion; the putting off of individual existence is the only true release. Other systems assert, in flat contradiction of this view, the eternal persistence of the human soul; a basis of multiple consciousness in the One or else a dependent but still separate entity, it is constant, real, imperishable.

Amidst these various and conflicting opinions the seeker of the Truth has to decide for himself which shall be for him the Knowledge. But if our aim is a spiritual release or a spiritual fulfilment, then the exceeding of this little mould of ego is imperative. In human egoism and its satisfaction there can be no divine culmination and deliverance. A certain purification from egoism is the condition even of ethical progress and elevation, for social good and perfection; much more is it indispensable for inner peace, purity and joy. But a much more radical deliverance, not only from egoism but from ego-idea and ego-sense, is needed if our aim is to raise human into divine nature. Experience shows that, in proportion as we deliver ourselves from the limiting mental and vital ego, we command a wider life, a larger existence, a higher consciousness, a happier soul-state, even a greater knowledge, power and scope. Even the aim which the most mundane philosophy pursues, the fulfilment, perfection, satisfaction of the individual, is best assured not by satisfying the narrow ego but by finding freedom in a higher and larger self. There is no happiness in smallness of the being, says the Scripture, it is with the large being that happiness comes. The ego is by its nature a smallness of being; it brings contraction of the consciousness and with the contraction limitation of knowledge, disabling ignorance,—confinement and a diminution of power and by that diminution incapacity and weakness,— scission of oneness and by that scission disharmony and failure of sympathy and love and understanding,—inhibition or fragmentation of delight of being and by that fragmentation pain and sorrow. To recover what is lost we must break out of the walls of ego. The ego must either disappear in impersonality or fuse into a larger I: it must fuse into the wider cosmic "I" which comprehends all these smaller selves or the transcendent of which even the cosmic self is a diminished image.

But this cosmic self is spiritual in essence and in experience; it must not be confused with the collective existence, with any group soul or the life and body of a human society or even of all mankind. The subordination of the ego to the progress and happiness of the human race is now a governing idea in the world's thought and ethics; but this is a mental and moral and not a spiritual ideal. For that progress is a series of constant mental, vital and physical vicissitudes, it has no firm spiritual content, and offers no sure standing-ground to the soul of man. The consciousness of collective humanity is only a larger comprehensive edition or a sum of individual egos. Made of the same substance, in the same mould of nature, it has not in it any greater light, any more eternal sense of itself, any purer source of peace, joy and deliverance. It is rather even more tortured, troubled and obscured, certainly more vague, confused and unprogressive. The individual is in this respect greater than the mass and cannot be called on to subordinate his more luminous possibilities to this darker entity. If light, peace, deliverance, a better state of existence are to come, they must descend into the soul from something wider than the individual, but also from something higher than the collective ego. Altruism, philanthropy, the service of mankind are in themselves mental or moral ideals, not laws of the spiritual life. If into the spiritual aim there enters the impulse to deny the personal self or to serve humanity or the world at large, it comes not from the ego nor from the collective sense of the race, but from something more occult and profound transcendent of both these things; for it is founded on a sense of the Divine in all and it works not for the sake of the ego or the race but for the sake of the Divine and its purpose in the person or group or collective. It is this transcendent Source which we must seek and serve, this vaster being and consciousness to which the race and the individual are minor terms of its existence.

There is indeed a truth behind the pragmatic impulse which an exclusive one-sided spirituality is apt to ignore or deny or belittle. It is this that since the individual and the universal are terms of that higher and vaster Being, their fulfilment must have some real place in the supreme Existence. There must be behind them some high purpose in the supreme Wisdom and Knowledge, some eternal strain in the supreme

Delight: they cannot have been, they were not created in vain. But the perfection and satisfaction of humanity like the perfection and satisfaction of the individual, can only be securely compassed and founded upon a more eternal yet unseized truth and right of things. Minor terms of some greater Existence, they can fulfil themselves only when that of which they are the terms is known and possessed. The greatest service to humanity, the surest foundation for its true progress, happiness and perfection is to prepare or find the way by which the individual and the collective man can transcend the ego and live in its true self, no longer bound to ignorance, incapacity, disharmony and sorrow. It is by the pursuit of the eternal and not by living bound in the slow collective evolution of Nature that we can best assure even that evolutionary, collective, altruistic aim our modern thought and idealism have set before us. But it is in itself a secondary aim; to find, know and possess the Divine existence, consciousness and nature and to live in it for the Divine is our true aim and the one perfection to which we must aspire.

It is then in the way of the spiritual philosophies and religions, not in that of any earth-bound materialistic doctrine, that the seeker of the highest knowledge has to walk, even if with enriched aims and a more comprehensive spiritual purpose. But how far has he to proceed in the elimination of the ego? In the ancient way of knowledge we arrive at the elimination of the ego-sense which attaches itself to the body, to the life, to the mind and says of all or any of them, "This is I". Not only do we, as in the way of works, get rid of the "I" of the worker and see the Lord alone as the true source of all works and sanction of works and His executive Nature-power or else His supreme Shakti as the sole agent and worker,—but we get rid also of the ego-sense which mistakes the instruments or the expressions of our being for our true self and spirit. But even if all this has been done, something remains still; there remains a substratum of all these, a general sense of the separate I. This substratum ego is something vague, indefinable, elusive; it does not or need not attach itself to anything in particular as the self; it does not identify itself with anything collective; it is a sort of fundamental form or power of the mind which compels the mental being to feel himself as a perhaps indefinable but still a limited being which is not mind, life or body, but under which their activities proceed in Nature. The others were a qualified ego-idea and ego-sense supporting themselves on the play of the Prakriti; but this is the pure fundamental ego-power supporting itself on the consciousness of the mental Purusha. And because it seems to be above or behind the play and not in it, because it does not say "I am the mind, life or body," but "I am a being on whom the action of mind, life and body depends," many think themselves released and mistake this elusive Ego for the One, the Divine, the true Purusha or at the very least for the true Person within them,—mistaking the indefinable for the Infinite. But so long as this fundamental ego-sense remains, there is no absolute release. The egoistic life, even if diminished in force and intensity, can still continue well enough with this support. If there is the error in identification, the ego life may under that pretext get rather an exaggerated intensity and force. Even if there is no much error, the ego life may be wider, purer, more flexible and release may be now much easier to attain and nearer to accomplishment, but still there is as yet no definitive release. It is imperative to go farther, to get rid of this indefinable but fundamental ego-sense also and get back to the Purusha on whom it is supporting itself, of whom it is a shadow; the shadow has to disappear and by its disappearance reveal the spirit's unclouded substance.

That substance is the self of the man called in European thought the Monad, in Indian philosophy, Jiva or Jivatman, the living entity, the self of the living creature. This Jiva is not the mental ego-sense constructed by the workings of Nature for her temporary purpose. It is not a thing bound, as the mental being, the vital, the physical are bound, by her habits, laws or processes. The Jiva is a spirit and self, superior to Nature. It is true that it consents to her acts, reflects her moods and upholds the triple medium of mind, life and body through which she casts them upon the soul's consciousness; but it is itself a living reflection or a soul-form or a self-creation of the Spirit universal and transcendent. The One Spirit who has mirrored some of His modes of being in the world and in the soul, is multiple in the Jiva. That Spirit is the very Self of our self, the One and the Highest, the Supreme we have to realise, the infinite existence into which we have to enter. And so far the teachers walk in company, all agreeing that this is the supreme object of knowledge, of works and of devotion, all agreeing that if it is to be attained, the Jiva must release himself from the ego-sense which belongs to the lower Nature or Maya. But here they part company and each goes his own way. The Monist fixes his feet on the path of an exclusive Knowledge and sets for us as sole ideal an entire return, loss, immersion or extinction of the Jiva in the Supreme. The Dualist or the partial Monist turns to the path of Devotion and directs us to shed indeed the lower ego and material life, but to see as the highest destiny of the spirit of man, not the self-annihilation of the Buddhist, not the self-immersion of the Adwaitin, not a swallowing up of the many by the One, but an eternal existence absorbed in the thought, love and enjoyment of the Supreme, the One, the All-Lover.

For the disciple of an integral Yoga there can be no hesitation; as a seeker of knowledge it is the integral knowledge and not anything either half-way and attractive or high-pinnacled and exclusive he must seek. He must soar to the utmost height, but also circle and spread to the most all-embracing wideness, not binding himself to any rigid structure of metaphysical thought, but free to admit and combine all the soul's highest and greatest and fullest and most numerous experiences. If the highest height of spiritual experience, the sheer summit of all realisation is the absolute union of the soul with the Transcendent who exceeds the individual and the universe, the widest scope of that union is the discovery of that very Transcendent as the source, support, continent, informing and constituent spirit and substance of both these manifesting powers of the divine Essence and the divine Nature. Whatever the path, this must be for him the goal. The Yoga of Action also is not fulfilled, is not absolute, is not victoriously complete until the seeker has felt and lives in his essential and integral oneness with the Supreme. One he must be with the Divine both in his highest and inmost and in his widest being and consciousness, in his work, his will, his power of action, his mind, body, life. Otherwise he is only released from the illusion of individual works, but not released from the illusion of separate being and instrumentality. As the servant and instrument of the Divine he works, but the crown of his labour and its perfect base or motive is oneness with that which he serves and fulfils. The Yoga of devotion too is complete only when the lover and the Beloved are unified and difference is abolished in the ecstasy of a divine oneness; and yet in the mystery of this unification there is the sole existence of the Beloved but no extinction or absorption of the lover. It is the highest unity which is the express direction of the path of knowledge, the call to absolute oneness is its impulse, the experience of it its magnet, but it is this very highest unity which takes as its field of manifestation in him the largest possible cosmic wideness. Obeying the necessity to withdraw successively from the practical egoism of our triple nature and its fundamental ego-sense, we come to the realisation of the spirit, the self, lord of this individual human manifestation, but our knowledge is not integral if we do not make this self in the individual one with the cosmic spirit and find their greater reality above in an inexpressible but not unknowable Transcendence. The Jiva, possessed of himself, must give himself up into the being of the Divine. The self of the man must be made one with the Self of all; the self of the finite individual must pour itself into the boundless finite and that cosmic spirit too must be exceeded in the transcendent Infinite.

This cannot be done without an uncompromising abolition of the ego-sense at its very basis and source. In the path of Knowledge one attempts this abolition, negatively by a denial of the reality of the ego, positively by a constant fixing of the thought upon the idea of the One and the Infinite in itself or the One and Infinite everywhere. This, if persistently done, changes in the end the mental outlook on oneself and the whole world and there is a kind of mental realisation; but afterwards by degrees or perhaps rapidly and imperatively and almost at the beginning the mental realisation deepens into spiritual experience— a realisation in the very substance of our being. More and more frequent conditions come of something indefinable and illimitable, a peace, a silence, a joy, a bliss beyond expression, a sense of absolute impersonal Power, a pure existence, a pure consciousness, an all-pervading Presence. The ego persists in itself or in its habitual movements, but the place of the one becomes more and more loosened, the others are broken, crushed, more and more rejected, becoming weak in their intensity, limp or mechanical in their action. In the end there is a constant giving up of the whole consciousness into the being of the Supreme. In the beginning when the restless confusion and obscuring impurity of our outward nature is active, when the mental, vital, physical ego-sense are still powerful, this new mental outlook, these experiences may be found difficult in the extreme: but once that triple egoism is discouraged or moribund and the instruments of the Spirit are set right and purified, in an entirely pure, silent, clarified, widened consciousness the purity, infinity, stillness of the One reflects itself like the sky in a limpid lake. A meeting or a taking in of the reflected Consciousness by that which reflects it becomes more and more pressing and possible; the bridging or abolition of the atmospheric gulf between that immutable ethereal impersonal vastness and this once mobile whirl or narrow stream of personal existence is no longer an arduous improbability and may be even a frequent experience, if not yet an entirely permanent state. For even before complete purification, if the strings of the egoistic heart and mind are already sufficiently frayed and loosened, the Jiva can by a sudden snapping of the main cords escape, ascending like a bird freed into the spaces or widening like a liberated flood into the One and Infinite. There is first a sudden sense of a cosmic consciousness, a casting of oneself into the universal; from that universality one can aspire more easily to the Transcendent. There is a pushing back and rending or a rushing down of the walls that imprisoned our conscious being; there is a loss of all sense of individuality and personality, of all placement in Space or Time or action and law of Nature; there is no longer an ego, a person definite and definable, but only consciousness, only existence, only peace or bliss; one becomes immortality, becomes eternity, becomes infinity. All that is left of the personal soul is a hymn of peace and freedom and bliss vibrating somewhere in the Eternal.

When there is an insufficient purity in the mental being, the release appears at first to be partial and temporary; the Jiva seems to descend again into the egoistic life and the higher consciousness to be withdrawn from him. In reality, what happens is that a cloud or veil intervenes between the lower nature and the higher consciousness and the Prakriti resumes for a time its old habit of working under the pressure but not always with a knowledge or present memory of that high experience. What works in it then is a ghost of the old ego supporting a mechanical repetition of the old habits upon the remnants of confusion and impurity still left in the system. The cloud intervenes and disappears, the rhythm of ascent and descent renews itself until the impurity has been worked out. This period of alternations may easily be long in the integral Yoga; for there an entire perfection of the system is required; it must be capable at all times and in all conditions and all circumstances, whether of action or inaction, of admitting and then living in the consciousness of the supreme Truth. Nor is it enough for the sadhaka to have the utter realisation only in the trance of Samadhi or in a motionless quietude, but he must in trance or in waking, in passive reflection or energy of action be able to remain in the constant Samadhi of the firmly founded Brahmic consciousness.[1] But if or when our conscious being has become sufficiently pure and clear, then there is a firm station in the higher consciousness. The impersonalised Jiva, one with the universal or possessed by the Transcendent, lives high-seated above[2] and looks down undisturbed at whatever remnants of the old working of Nature may revisit the system. He cannot be moved by the workings of the three modes of Prakriti in his lower being, nor can he be shaken from his station by the attacks even of grief and suffering. And finally, there being no veil between, the higher peace overpowers the lower disturbance and mobility. There is a settled silence in which the soul can take sovereign possession of itself above and below and altogether.

Such possession is not indeed the aim of the traditional Yoga of knowledge whose object is rather to get away from the above and the below and the all into the indefinable Absolute. But whatever the aim, the path of knowledge must lead to one first result, an absolute quietude; for unless the old action of Nature in us be entirely quieted, it is difficult if not impossible to found either any true soul-status or any divine activity. Our nature acts on a basis of confusion and restless compulsion to action, the Divine acts freely out of a fathomless calm. Into that abyss of tranquillity we must plunge and become that, if we are to annul the hold of this lower nature upon the soul. Therefore the universalised Jiva first ascends into the Silence; it becomes vast, tranquil, actionless. What action takes place, whether of body and these organs or any working whatever, the Jiva sees but does not take part in, authorise or in any way associate itself with it. There is action, but no personal actor, no bondage, no responsibility. If personal action is needed, then the Jiva has to keep or recover what has been called the form of the ego, a sort of mental image of an "I" that is the knower, devotee, servant or instrument, but an image only and not a reality. If even that is not there, still action can continue by the mere continued force of Prakriti, without any personal actor, without indeed there being any sense of an actor at all; for the Self into which the Jiva has cast its being is the actionless, the fathomlessly still. The path of works leads to the realisation of the Lord, but here even the Lord is not known; there is only the silent Self and Prakriti doing her works, even, as it seems at first, not with truly living entities but with names and forms existing in the Self but which the Self does not admit as real. The soul may go even beyond this realisation; it may either rise to the Brahman on the other side of all idea of Self as a Void of everything that is here, a Void of unnameable peace and extinction of all, even of the Sat, even of that Existent which is the impersonal basis of individual or universal personality; or else it may unite with it as an ineffable "That" of which nothing can be said; for the universe and all that is does not even exist in That, but appears to the mind as a dream more unsubstantial than any dream ever seen or imagined, so that even the word dream seems too positive a thing to express its entire unreality. These experiences are the foundation of that lofty Illusionism which takes such firm hold of the human mind in its highest overleapings of itself.

These ideas of dream and illusion are simply results in our still existent mentality of the new poise of the Jiva and its denial of the claim made upon it by its old mental associations and view of life and existence. In reality, the Prakriti does not act for itself or by its own motion, but with the Self as lord; for out of that Silence wells all this action, that apparent Void looses out as if into movement all these infinite riches of experience. To this realisation the sadhaka of the integral Yoga must arrive by the process that we shall hereafter describe. What then, when he so resumes his hold upon the universe and views no longer himself in the world but the cosmos in himself, will be the position of the Jiva or what will fill in his new consciousness the part of the ego-sense? There will be no ego-sense even if there is a sort of individualisation for the purposes of the play of universal consciousness in an individual mind and frame; and for this reason that all will be unforgettably the One and every Person or Purusha will be to him the One in many forms or rather in many aspects and poises, Brahman acting upon Brahman, one Nara-Narayana[3] everywhere. In that larger play of the Divine the joy of the relations of divine love also is possible without the lapse into the ego-sense,—just as the supreme state of human love likewise is described as the unity of one soul in two bodies. The ego-sense is not indispensable to the world-play in which it is so active and so falsifies the truth of things; the truth is always the One at work on itself, at play with itself, infinite in unity, infinite in multiplicity. When the individualised consciousness rises to and lives in that truth of the cosmic play, then even in full action, even in possession of the lower being the Jiva remains still one with the Lord, and there is no bondage and no delusion. He is in possession of Self and released from the ego.

---

1. Gita.
2. *Udāsīna*, the word for the spiritual "indifference", that is to say the unattached freedom of the soul touched by the supreme knowledge.
3. The Divine, Narayana, making itself one with humanity even as the human, Nara becomes one with the Divine.

# THE REALISATION OF THE COSMIC SELF

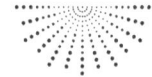

OUR FIRST imperative aim when we draw back from mind, life, body and all else that is not our eternal being, is to get rid of the false idea of self by which we identify ourselves with the lower existence and can realise only our apparent being as perishable or mutable creatures in a perishable or ever mutable world. We have to know ourselves as the self, the spirit, the eternal; we have to exist consciously in our true being. Therefore this must be our primary, if not our first one and all-absorbing idea and effort in the path of knowledge. But when we have realised the eternal self that we are, when we have become that inalienably, we have still a secondary aim, to establish the true relation between this eternal self that we are and the mutable existence and mutable world which till now we had falsely taken for our real being and our sole possible status.

In order that there should be any real relation, it must be a relation between two realities. Formerly we had thought the eternal self to be a remote concept far from our mundane existence if not an illusion and an unreality, because in the nature of things we could not conceive of ourselves as anything except this mind, life, body, changing and moving in the succession of Time. When we have once got rid of our confinement to this lower status, we are apt to seize on the other side of the same erroneous relation between self and world; we tend to regard this eternity which we increasingly are or in which we live as the sole reality and begin to look down from it upon the world and man as a remote illusion and unreality, because that is a status quite opposite to our new foundation in which we no longer place our roots of consciousness, from which we have been lifted up and transfigured and with which we seem to have no longer any binding link. Especially is this likely to happen if we have made the finding of the eternal Self not only our primary, but our one and absorbing objective in the withdrawal from the lower triplicity; for then we are likely to shoot at once from pure mind to pure spirit without treading the stairs between this middle and that summit and we tend to fix on our consciousness the profound sense of a gulf which we cannot bridge and can no longer cross over again except by a painful fall.

But the self and the world are in an eternal close relation and there is a connection between them, not a gulf that has to be overleaped. Spirit and material existence are highest and lowest rung of an orderly and progressive series. Therefore between the two there must be a real relation and principle of connection by which the eternal Brahman is able to be at once pure Spirit and Self and yet hold in himself the universe of himself; and it must be possible for the soul that is one with or in union with the Eternal to adopt the same poise of divine relation in place of our present ignorant immersion in the world. This principle of connection is the eternal unity between the Self and all existences; of that eternal unity the liberated soul must be capable, just as the ever free and unbound Divine is capable of it, and that we should realise equally with the pure self-existence at which we have first to aim. For integral self-possession we must be one not only with the Self, with God, but with all existences. We must take back in the right relation and in the poise of an eternal Truth the world of our manifested existence peopled by our fellow-beings from which we had drawn back because we were bound to them in a wrong relation and in the poise of a falsehood created in Time by the principle of divided consciousness with all its oppositions, discords and dualities. We have to take back all things and beings into our new consciousness but as one with all, not divided from them by an egoistic individuality.

In other words, besides the consciousness of the transcendent Self pure, self-existent, timeless, spaceless we have to accept and become the cosmic consciousness, we have to identify our being with the Infinite who makes himself the base and continent of the worlds and dwells in all existences. This is the realisation which the ancient Vedantins spoke of as seeing all existences in the self and the self in all existences; and in addition they speak of the crowning realisation of the man in whom the original miracle of existence has been repeated, self-being has become all these existences that belong to the worlds of the becoming.[1] In these three terms is expressed, fundamentally, the whole of that real relation between the self and the world which we have to substitute for the false relation created by the limiting ego. This is the new vision and sense of infinite being which we have to acquire, this the foundation of that unity with all which we have to establish.

For our real self is not the individual mental being, that is only a figure, an appearance; our real self is cosmic, infinite, it is one with all existence and the inhabitant of all existences. The self behind our mind, life and body is the same as the self behind the mind, life and body of all our fellow-beings, and if we come to possess it, we shall naturally, when we turn to look out again upon them, tend to become one with them in the common basis of our consciousness. It is true that the mind opposes any such identification and if we allow it to persist in its old habits and activities, it will rather strive to bring again its veil of dissonances over our new realisation and possession of self than to shape and subject itself to this true and eternal vision of things. But in the first place, if we have proceeded rightly on the path of our Yoga, we shall have attained to Self through a purified mind and heart, and a purified mind is one that is necessarily passive and open to the knowledge. Secondly even the mind in spite of its tendency to limit and divide can be taught to think in the rhythm of the unifying Truth instead of the broken terms of the limiting appearance. We must therefore accustom it by meditation and concentration to cease to think of things and beings as separately existent in themselves and rather to think always of the One everywhere and of all things as the One. Although we have spoken hitherto of the withdrawing motion of the Jiva as the first necessity of knowledge and as if it were to be pursued alone and by itself, yet in fact it is better for the sadhaka of the integral Yoga to unite the two movements. By one he will find the self within, by the other he will find that self in all that seems to us at present to be outside us. It is possible indeed to begin with the latter movement, to realise all things in this visible and sensible existence as God or Brahman or Virat Purusha and then to go beyond to all that is behind the Virat. But this has its inconveniences and it is better, if that be found possible, to combine the two movements.

This realisation of all things as God or Brahman has, as we have seen, three aspects of which we can conveniently make three successive stages of experience. First, there is the Self in whom all beings exist. The Spirit, the Divine has manifested itself as infinite self-extended being, self-existent, pure, not subject to Time and Space, but supporting Time and Space as figures of its consciousness. It is more than all things and contains them all within that self-extended being and consciousness, not bound by anything that it creates, holds or becomes, but free and infinite and all-blissful. It holds them, in the old image, as the infinite ether contains in itself all objects. This image of the ethereal (Akasha) Brahman may indeed be of great practical help to the sadhaka who finds a difficulty in meditating on what seems to him at first an abstract and unseizable idea. In the image of the ether, not physical but an encompassing ether of vast being, consciousness and bliss, he may seek to see with the mind and to feel in his mental being this supreme existence and to identify it in oneness with the self within him. By such meditation the mind may be brought to a favourable state of predisposition in which, by the rending or withdrawing of the veil, the supramental vision may flood the mentality and change entirely all our seeing. And upon that change of seeing, as it becomes more and more potent and insistent and occupies all our consciousness, there will supervene eventually a change of becoming so that what we see we become. We shall be in our self-consciousness not so much cosmic as ultra-cosmic, infinite. Mind and life and body will then be only movements in that infinity which we have become, and we shall see that what exists is not world at all but simply this infinity of spirit in which move the mighty cosmic harmonies of its own images of self-conscious becoming.

But what then of all these forms and existences that make up the harmony? Shall they be to us only images, empty name and form without any informing reality, poor worthless things in themselves and however grandiose, puissant or beautiful they once seemed to our mental vision, now to be rejected and held of no value? Not so; although that would be the first natural result of a very intense absorption in the infinity of the all-containing Self to the exclusion of the infinities that it contains. But these things are not empty, not mere unreal name and form imagined by a cosmic Mind; they are, as we have said, in their reality self-conscious becomings of the Self, that is to say, the Self dwells within all of them even as within us, conscious of them, governing their motion, blissful in his habitation as in his embrace of all that he becomes. As the ether both contains and is as it were contained in the jar, so this Self both contains and inhabits all existences, not in a physical but in a spiritual sense, and is their reality. This indwelling State of the Self we have to realise; we have to see and ourselves to become in our consciousness the Self in all existences. We have, putting aside all vain resistance of the intellect and the mental associations, to know that the Divine inhabits all these becomings and is their true Self and conscious Spirit, and not to know it only intellectually but to know by a self-experience that shall compel into its own diviner mould all the habits of the mental consciousness.

This Self that we are has finally to become to our self-consciousness entirely one with all existences in spite of its exceeding them. We have to see it not only as that which contains and inhabits all, but that which is all, not only as indwelling spirit, but also as the name and form, the movement and the master of the movement, the mind and life and body. It is by this final realisation that we shall resume entirely in the right poise and the vision of the Truth all that we drew back from in the first movement of recoil and withdrawal. The individual mind, life and body which we recoiled from as not our true being, we shall recover as a true becoming of the Self, but no longer in a purely individual narrowness. We shall take up the mind not as a separate mentality imprisoned in a petty motion, but as a large movement of the universal mind, the life not as an egoistic activity of vitality and sensation and desire, but as a free movement of the universal life, the body not as a physical prison of the soul but as a subordinate instrument and detachable robe, realising that also as a movement of universal Matter, a cell of the cosmic Body. We shall come to feel all the consciousness of the physical world as one with our physical consciousness, feel all the energies of the cosmic life around as our own energies, feel all the heart-beats of the great cosmic impulse and seeking in our heart-beats set to the rhythm of the divine Ananda, feel all the action of the universal mind flowing into our mentality and our thought-action flowing out upon it as a wave into that wide sea. This unity embracing all mind, life and matter in the light of a supramental Truth and the pulse of a spiritual Bliss will be to us our internal fulfilment of the Divine in a complete cosmic consciousness.

But since we must embrace all this in the double term of the Being and the Becoming, the knowledge that we shall possess must be complete and integral. It must not stop with the realisation of the pure

Self and Spirit, but include also all those modes of the Spirit by which it supports, develops and throws itself out into its cosmic manifestation. Self-knowledge and world-knowledge must be made one in the all-ensphering knowledge of the Brahman.

---

1. Isha Upanishad.

# THE MODES OF THE SELF

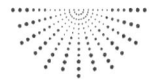

SINCE the Self which we come to realise by the path of knowledge is not only the reality which lies behind and supports the states and movements of our psychological being, but also that transcendent and universal Existence which has manifested itself in all the movements of the universal, the knowledge of the Self includes also the knowledge of the principles of Being, its fundamental modes and its relations with the principles of the phenomenal universe. This was what was meant by the Upanishad when it spoke of the Brahman as that which being known all is known.[1] It has to be realised first as the pure principle of Existence, afterwards, says the Upanishad, its essential modes become clear to the soul which realises it. We may indeed, before realisation, try to analyse by the metaphysical reason and even understand intellectually what Being is and what the world is, but such metaphysical understanding is not the Knowledge. Moreover, we may have the realisation in knowledge and vision, but this is incomplete without realisation in the entire soul-experience and the unity of all our being with that which we realise.[2] It is the science of Yoga to know and the art of Yoga to be unified with the Highest so that we may live in the Self and act from that supreme poise, becoming one not only in the conscious essence but in the conscious law of our being with the transcendent Divine whom all things and creatures, whether ignorantly or with partial knowledge and experience, seek to express through the lower law of their members. To know the highest Truth and to be in harmony with it is the condition of right being, to express it in all that we are, experience and do is the condition of right living. But rightly to know and express the Highest is not easy for man the mental being because the highest Truth and therefore the highest modes of existence are supramental. They repose on the essential unity of what seem to the intellect and mind and are to our mental experience of the world opposite poles of existence and idea and therefore irreconcilable opposites and contradictions, but to the supramental experience are complementary aspects of the same Truth. We have seen this already in the necessity of realising the Self as at once one and many; for we have to realise each thing and being as That; we have to realise the unity of all as That, both in the unity of sum and in the oneness of essence; and we have to realise That as the Transcendent who is beyond all this unity and this multiplicity which we see everywhere as the two opposite, yet companion poles of all existence. For every individual being is the Self, the Divine in spite of the outward limitations of the mental and physical form through which it presents itself at the actual moment, in the actual field of space, in the actual succession of circumstances that make up the web of inner state and outward action and event through which we know the individual. So, equally, every collectivity small or great is each the Self, the Divine similarly expressing itself in the conditions of this manifestation. We cannot really know any individual or any collectivity if we know it only as it appears inwardly to itself or outwardly to us, but only if we know it as the Divine, the One, our own Self employing its various essential modes and its occasional circumstances of self-manifestation. Until we have transformed the habits of our mentality so that it shall live entirely in this knowledge reconciling all differences in the One, we do not live in the real Truth, because we do not live in the real Unity. The accomplished sense of Unity is not that in which all are regarded as parts of one whole, waves of one sea, but that in which each as well as the All is regarded wholly as the Divine, wholly as our Self in a supreme identity.

And yet, so complex is the Maya of the Infinite, there is a sense in which the view of all as parts of the whole, waves of the sea or even as in a sense separate entities becomes a necessary part of the integral Truth and the integral Knowledge. For if the Self is always one in all, yet we see that for the purposes at least of the cyclic manifestation it expresses itself in perpetual soul-forms which preside over the movements of our personality through the worlds and the aeons. This persistent soul-existence is the real Individuality which stands behind the constant mutations of the thing we call our personality. It is not a limited ego but a thing in itself infinite; it is in truth the Infinite itself consenting from one plane of its being to reflect itself in a perpetual soul-experience. This is the truth which underlies the Sankhya theory of many Purushas, many essential, infinite, free and impersonal souls reflecting the movements of a single cosmic energy. It stands also, in a different way, behind the very different philosophy of qualified Monism which arose as a protest against the metaphysical excesses of Buddhistic Nihilism and illusionist Adwaita. The old semi-Buddhistic, semi-Sankhya theory which saw only the Quiescent and nothing else in the world except a constant combination of the five elements and the three modes of inconscient Energy lighting up their false activity by the consciousness of the Quiescent in which it is reflected, is not the whole truth of the Brahman. We are not a mere mass of changing mind-stuff, life-stuff, body-stuff taking different forms of mind and life and body from birth to birth, so that at no time is there any real self or conscious reason of existence behind all the flux or none except that Quiescent who cares for none of these things. There is a real and stable power of our being behind the constant mutation of our mental, vital and physical personality, and this we have to know and preserve in order that the Infinite may manifest Himself through it according to His will in whatever range and for whatever purpose of His eternal cosmic activity.

And if we regard existence from the standpoint of the possible eternal and infinite relations of this One from whom all things proceed, these Many of whom the One is the essence and the origin and this Energy, Power, or Nature through which the relations of the One and the Many are maintained, we shall see a certain justification even for the dualist philosophies and religions which seem to deny most energetically the unity of beings and to make an unbridgeable differentiation between the Lord and His creatures. If in their grosser forms these religions aim only at the ignorant joys of the lower heavens, yet there is a far higher and profounder sense in which we may appreciate the cry of the devotee poet when in a homely and vigorous metaphor he claimed the right of the soul to enjoy for ever the ecstasy of its embrace of the Supreme. "I do not want to become sugar," he wrote, "I want to eat sugar." However strongly we may found ourselves on the essential identity of the one Self in all, we need not regard that cry as the mere aspiration of a certain kind of spiritual sensuousness or the rejection by an attached and ignorant soul of the pure and high austerity of the supreme Truth. On the contrary, it aims in its positive part at a deep and mysterious truth of Being which no human language can utter, of which human reason can give no adequate account, to which the heart has the key and which no pride of the soul of knowledge insisting on its own pure austerity can abolish. But that belongs properly to the summit of the path of Devotion and there we shall have again to return to it.

The sadhaka of an integral Yoga will take an integral view of his goal and seek its integral realisation. The Divine has many essential modes of His eternal self-manifestation, possesses and finds Himself on many planes and through many poles of His being; to each mode its purpose, to each plane or pole its fulfilment both in the apex and the supreme scope of the eternal Unity. It is necessarily through the individual Self that we must arrive at the One, for that is the basis of all our experience. By Knowledge we arrive at identity with the One; for there is, in spite of the Dualist, an essential identity by which we can plunge into our Source and free ourselves from all bondage to individuality and even from all bondage to universality. Nor is the experience of that identity a gain for knowledge only or for the pure state of abstract being. The height of all our action also, we have seen, is the immersion of ourselves in the Lord through unity with the divine Will or Conscious-Power by the way of works; the height of love is the rapturous immersion of ourselves in unity of ecstatic delight with the object of our love and adoration. But again for divine works in the world the individual Self converts itself into a centre of consciousness through which the divine Will, one with the divine Love and Light, pours itself out in the multiplicity of the universe. We arrive in the same way at our unity with all our fellow-beings through the identity of this self with the Supreme and with the self in all others. At the same time in the action of Nature we preserve by it as soul-form of the One a differentiation which enables us to preserve relations of difference in Oneness with other beings and with the Supreme Himself. The relations will necessarily be very different in essence and spirit from those which we had when we lived entirely in the Ignorance and Oneness was a mere name or a struggling aspiration of imperfect love, sympathy or yearning. Unity will be the law, difference will be simply for the various enjoyment of that unity. Neither descending again into that plane of division which clings to the separation of the ego-sense nor attached to an exclusive seeking for pure identity which cannot have to do with any play of difference, we shall embrace and reconcile the two poles of being where they meet in the infinity of the Highest.

The Self, even the individual self, is different from our personality as it is different from our mental ego-sense. Our personality is never the same; it is a constant mutation and various combination. It is not a basic consciousness, but a development of forms of consciousness,—not a power of being, but a various play of partial powers of being,—not the enjoyer of the self-delight of our existence, but a seeking after various notes and tones of experience which shall more or less render that delight in the mutability of relations. This also is Purusha and Brahman, but it is the mutable Purusha, the phenomenon of the Eternal, not its stable reality. The Gita makes a distinction between three Purushas who constitute the whole state and action of the divine Being, the Mutable, the Immutable and the Highest which is beyond and embraces the other two. That Highest is the Lord in whom we have to live, the supreme Self in us and in all. The Immutable is the silent, actionless, equal, unchanging self which we reach when we draw back from activity to passivity, from the play of consciousness and force and the seeking of delight to the pure and constant basis of consciousness and force and delight through which the Highest, free, secure and unattached, possesses and enjoys the play. The Mutable is the substance and immediate motive of that changing flux of personality through which the relations of our cosmic life are made possible. The mental being fixed in the Mutable moves in its flux and has not possession of an eternal peace and power and self-delight; the soul fixed in the Immutable holds all these in itself but cannot act in the world; but the soul that can live in the Highest enjoys the eternal peace and power and delight and wideness of being, is not bound in its self-knowledge and self-power by character and personality or by forms of its force and habits of its consciousness and yet uses them all with a large freedom and power for the self-expression of the Divine in the world. Here again the change is not any alteration of the essential modes of the Self, but consists in our emergence into the freedom of the Highest and the right use of the divine law of our being.

Connected with this triple mode of the Self is that distinction which Indian philosophy has drawn between the Qualitied and the Qualitiless Brahman and European thought has made between the Personal and the Impersonal God. The Upanishad indicates clearly enough the relative nature of this opposition, when it speaks of the Supreme as the "Qualitied who is without qualities".[3] We have again two essential modes, two fundamental aspects, two poles of eternal being, both of them exceeded in the transcendent divine Reality. They correspond practically to the Silent and the Active Brahman. For the whole action of the universe may be regarded from a certain point of view as the expression and shaping out in various ways of the numberless and infinite qualities of the Brahman. His being assumes by conscious Will all kinds of properties, shapings of the stuff of conscious being, habits as it were of cosmic character and power of dynamic self-consciousness, *guṇas*, into which all the cosmic action can be resolved. But by none of these nor by all of them nor by their utmost infinite potentiality is He bound; He is above all His qualities and on a certain plane of being rests free from them. The Nirguna or Unqualitied is not incapable of qualities, rather it is this very Nirguna or No-Quality who manifests Himself as Saguna, as Anantaguna, infinite quality, since He contains all in His absolute capacity of boundlessly varied self-revelation. He is free from them in the sense of exceeding them; and indeed if He were not free from them they could not be infinite; God would be subject to His qualities, bound by His nature, Prakriti would be supreme and Purusha its creation and plaything. The Eternal is bound neither by quality nor absence of quality, neither by Personality nor by Impersonality; He is Himself, beyond all our positive and all our negative definitions.

But if we cannot define the Eternal, we can unify ourselves with it. It has been said that we can become the Impersonal, but not the personal God, but this is only true in the sense that no one can become individually the Lord of all the universes; we *can* free ourselves into the existence of the active Brahman as well as that of the Silence; we can live in both, go back to our being in both, but each in its proper way, by becoming one with the Nirguna in our essence and one with the Saguna in the liberty of our active being, in our nature.[4] The Supreme pours Himself out of an eternal peace, poise and silence into an eternal activity, free and infinite, freely fixing for itself its self-determinations, using infinite quality to shape out of it varied combination of quality. We have to go back to that peace, poise and silence and act out of it with the divine freedom from the bondage of qualities but still using qualities even the most opposite largely and flexibly for the divine work in the world. Only, while the Lord acts out of the centre of all things, we have to act by transmission of His will and power and self-knowledge through the individual centre, the soul-form of Him which we are. The Lord is subject to nothing; the individual soul-form is subject to its own highest Self and the greater and more absolute is that subjection, the greater becomes its sense of absolute force and freedom.

The distinction between the Personal and the Impersonal is substantially the same as the Indian distinction, but the associations of the English words carry within them a certain limitation which is foreign to Indian thought. The personal God of the European religions is a Person in the human sense of the word, limited by His qualities though otherwise possessed of omnipotence and omniscience; it answers to the Indian special conceptions of Shiva or Vishnu or Brahma or of the Divine Mother of all, Durga or Kali. Each religion really erects a different personal Deity according to its own heart and thought to adore and serve. The fierce and inexorable God of Calvin is a different being from the sweet and loving God of St. Francis, as the gracious Vishnu is different from the terrible though always loving and beneficent Kali who has pity even in her slaying and saves by her destructions. Shiva, the God of ascetic renunciation who destroys all things seems to be a different being from Vishnu and Brahma, who act by grace, love, preservation of the creature or for life and creation. It is obvious that such conceptions can be only in a very partial and relative sense true descriptions of the infinite and omnipresent Creator and Ruler of the universe. Nor does Indian religious thought affirm them as adequate descriptions. The Personal God is not limited by His qualities, He is Ananta-guna, capable of infinite qualities and beyond them and lord of them to use them as He will, and He manifests Himself in various names and forms of His infinite godhead to satisfy the desire and need of the individual soul according to its own nature and personality. It is for this reason that the normal European mind finds it so difficult to understand Indian religion as distinct from Vedantic or Sankhya philosophy, because it cannot easily conceive of a personal God with infinite qualities, a personal God who is not a Person, but the sole real Person and the source of all personality. Yet that is the only valid and complete truth of the divine Personality.

The place of the divine Personality in our synthesis will best be considered when we come to speak of the Yoga of devotion; it is enough here to indicate that it has its place and keeps it in the integral Yoga even when liberation has been attained. There are practically three grades of the approach to the personal Deity; the first in which He is conceived with a particular form or particular qualities as the name and form of the Godhead which our nature and personality prefers;[5] a second in which

He is the one real Person, the All-Personality, the Ananta-guna; a third in which we get back to the ultimate source of all idea and fact of personality in that which the Upanishad indicates by the single word *He* without fixing any attributes. It is there that our realisations of the personal and the impersonal Divine meet and become one in the utter Godhead. For the impersonal Divine is not ultimately an abstraction or a mere principle or a mere state or power and degree of being any more than we our-selves are really such abstractions. The intellect first approaches it through such conceptions, but realisation ends by exceeding them. Through the realisation of higher and higher principles of being and states of conscious existence we arrive not at the annullation of all in a sort of positive zero or even an inexpressible state of existence, but at the transcendent Existence itself which is also the Existent who transcends all definition by personality and yet is always that which is the essence of personality.

When in That we live and have our being, we can possess it in both its modes, the Impersonal in a supreme state of being and consciousness, in an infinite impersonality of self-possessing power and bliss, the Personal by the divine nature acting through the individual soul-form and by the relation between that and its transcendent and universal Self. We may keep even our relation with the personal Deity in His forms and names; if, for instance, our work is predominantly a work of Love it is as the Lord of Love that we can seek to serve and express Him, but we shall have at the same time an integral realisation of Him in all His names and forms and qualities and not mistake the front of Him which is prominent in our attitude to the world for all the infinite Godhead.

---

1. *yasmin vijñāte sarvaṁ vijñātam.*
2. This is the distinction made in the Gita between Sankhya and Yoga ; both are necessary to an integral knowledge.
3. *nirguṇo guṇī.*
4. *sādharmya-mukti.*
5. *iṣṭa-devatā.*

# THE REALISATION OF SACHCHIDANANDA

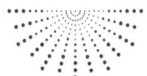

THE MODES of the Self which we have dealt with in our last Chapter may seem at first to be of a highly metaphysical character, to be intellectual conceptions more fit for philosophical analysis than for practical realisation. But this is a false distinction made by the division of our faculties. It is at least a fundamental principle of the ancient wisdom, the wisdom of the East on which we are founding ourselves, that philosophy ought not to be merely a lofty intellectual pastime or a play of dialectical subtlety or even a pursuit of metaphysical truth for its own sake, but a discovery by all right means of the basic truths of all-existence which ought then to become the guiding principles of our own existence. Sankhya, the abstract and analytical realisation of truth, is one side of Knowledge. Yoga, the concrete and synthetic realisation of it in our experience, inner state, outer life is the other. Both are means by which man can escape out of falsehood and ignorance and live in and by the truth. And since it is always the highest he can know or be capable of that must be the aim of the thinking man, it is the highest truth which the soul must seek out by thought and by life accomplish.

Here lies the whole importance of the part of the Yoga of Knowledge which we are now considering, the knowledge[1] of those essential principles of Being, those essential modes of self-existence on which the absolute Divine has based its self-manifestation. If the truth of our being is an infinite unity in which alone there is perfect wideness, light, knowledge, power, bliss, and if all our subjection to darkness, ignorance, weakness, sorrow, limitation comes of our viewing existence as a clash of infinitely multiple separate existences, then obviously it is the most practical and concrete and utilitarian as well as the most lofty and philosophical wisdom to find a means by which we can get away from the error and learn to live in the truth. So also, if that One is in its nature a freedom from bondage to this play of qualities which constitute our psychology and if from subjection to that play are born the struggle and discord in which we live, floundering eternally between the two poles of good and evil, virtue and sin, satisfaction and failure, joy and grief, pleasure and pain, then to get beyond the qualities and take our foundation in the settled peace of that which is always beyond them is the only practical wisdom. If attachment to mutable personality is the cause of our self-ignorance, of our discord and quarrel with ourself and with life and with others, and if there is an impersonal One in which no such discord and ignorance and vain and noisy effort exist because it is in eternal identity and harmony with itself, then to arrive in our souls at that impersonality and untroubled oneness of being is the one line and object of human effort to which our reason can consent to give the name of practicality.

There is such a unity, impersonality, freedom from the play of qualities which lifts us above the strife and surge of Nature in her eternal seeking through mind and body for the true key and secret of all her relations. And it is the ancient highest experience of mankind that only by arriving there, only by making oneself impersonal, one, still, self-gathered, superior to the mental and vital existence in that which is eternally superior to it, can a settled, because self-existent peace and internal freedom be acquired. Therefore this is the first, in a sense the characteristic and essential object of the Yoga of Knowledge. But, as we have insisted, this, if first, is not all; if the essential, it is not the complete object. Knowledge is not complete if it merely shows us how to get away from relations to that which is beyond relations, from personality to impersonality, from multiplicity to featureless unity. It must give us also that key, that secret of the whole play of relations, the whole variation of multiplicity, the whole clash and interaction of personalities for which cosmic existence is seeking. And knowledge is still incomplete if it gives us only an idea and cannot verify it in experience; we seek the key, the secret in order that we may govern the phenomenon by the reality it represents, heal its discords by the hidden principle of concord and unification behind them and arrive from the converging and diverging effort of the world to the harmony of its fulfilment. Not merely peace, but fulfilment is what the heart of the world is seeking and what a perfect and effective self-knowledge must give to it; peace can only be the eternal support, the infinite condition, the natural atmosphere of self-fulfilment.

Moreover, the knowledge that finds the true secret of multiplicity, personality, quality, play of relations, must show us some real oneness in essence of being and intimate unity in power of being between the impersonal and the source of personality, the qualitiless and that which expresses itself in qualities, the unity of existence and its many-featured multiplicity. The knowledge that leaves a yawning gulf between the two, can be no ultimate knowledge, however logical it may seem to the analytical intellect or however satisfactory to a self-dividing experience. True knowledge must arrive at a oneness which embraces even though it exceeds the totality of things, not at a oneness which is incapable of it and rejects it. For there can be no such original unbridgeable chasm of duality either in the All-existence itself or between any transcendent Oneness and the All-existent. And as in knowledge, so in experience and self-fulfilment. The experience which finds at the summit of things such an original unbridgeable chasm between two contrary principles and can at most succeed in overleaping it so that it has to live in one or the other, but cannot embrace and unify, is not the ultimate experience. Whether we seek to know by thought or by the vision of knowledge which surpasses thought or by that perfect self-experience in our own being which is the crown and fulfilment of realisation by knowledge, we must be able to think out, see, experience and live the all-satisfying unity. This is what we find in the conception, vision and experience of the One whose oneness does not cease or disappear from view by self-expression in the Many, who is free from bondage to qualities but is yet infinite quality, who contains and combines all relations, yet is ever absolute, who is no one person and yet all persons because He is all being and the one conscious Being. For the individual centre we call ourselves, to enter by its consciousness into this Divine and reproduce its nature in itself is the high and marvellous, yet perfectly rational and most supremely pragmatic and utilitarian goal before us. It is the fulfilment of our self-existence and at the same time the fulfilment of our cosmic existence, of the individual in himself and of the individual in his relation to the cosmic Many. Between these two terms there is no irreconcilable opposition: rather, our own self and the self of the cosmos having been discovered to be one, there must be between them an intimate unity.

In fact all these opposite terms are merely general conditions for the manifestation of conscious being in that Transcendent who is always one not only behind, but within all conditions however apparently opposite. And the original unifying spirit-stuff of them all and the one substantial mode of them all is that which has been described for the convenience of our thought as the trinity of Sachchidananda. Existence, Consciousness, Bliss, these are everywhere the three inseparable divine terms. None of them is really separate, though our mind and our mental experience can make not only the distinction, but the separation. Mind can say and think "I was, but unconscious"—for no being can say "I am, but unconscious"—and it can think and feel "I am, but miserable and without any pleasure in existence." In reality this is impossible. The existence we really are, the eternal "I am", of which it can never be true to say "It was", is nowhere and at no time unconscious. What we call unconsciousness is simply other-consciousness; it is the going in of this surface wave of our mental awareness of outer objects into our subliminal self-awareness and into our awareness too of other planes of existence. We are really no more unconscious when we are asleep or stunned or drugged or "dead" or in any other state, than when we are plunged in inner thought oblivious of our physical selves and our surroundings. For anyone who has advanced even a little way in Yoga, this is a most elementary proposition and one which offers no difficulty whatever to the thought because it is proved at every point by experience. It is more difficult to realise that existence and undelight of existence cannot go together. What we call misery, grief, pain, absence of delight is again merely a surface wave of the delight of existence which takes on to our mental experience these apparently opposite tints because of a certain trick of false reception in our divided being—which is not our existence at all but only a fragmentary formulation or discoloured spray of conscious-force tossed up by the infinite sea of our self-existence. In order to realise this we have to get away from our absorption in these surface habits, these petty tricks of our mental being,—and when we do get behind and away from them it is surprising how superficial they are, what ridiculously weak and little-penetrating pin-pricks they prove to be,—and we have to realise true existence, and true consciousness, and true experience of existence and consciousness, Sat, Chit and Ananda.

Chit, the divine Consciousness, is not our mental self-awareness; that we shall find to be only a form, a lower and limited mode or movement. As we progress and awaken to the soul in us and things, we shall realise that there is a consciousness also in the plant, in the metal, in the atom, in electricity, in everything that belongs to physical nature; we shall find even that it is not really in all respects a lower or more limited mode than the mental, on the contrary it is in many "inanimate" forms more intense, rapid, poignant, though less evolved towards the surface. But this also, this consciousness of vital and physical Nature is, compared with Chit, a lower and therefore a limited form, mode and movement. These lower modes of consciousness are the conscious-stuff of inferior planes in one indivisible existence. In ourselves also there is in our subconscious being an action which is precisely that of the "inanimate" physical Nature whence has been constituted the basis of our physical being, another which is that of plant-life, and another which is that of the lower animal creation around us. All these are so much dominated and conditioned by the thinking and reasoning conscious-being in us that we have no real awareness of these lower planes; we are unable to perceive in their own terms what these parts of us are doing, and receive it very imperfectly in the terms and values of the thinking and reasoning mind. Still we know well enough that there is an animal in us as well as that which is characteristically human,—something which is a creature of conscious instinct and impulse, not reflective or rational, as well as that which turns back in thought and will on its experience, meets it from above with the light and force of a higher plane and to some degree controls, uses and modifies it. But the animal in man is only the head of our subhuman being; below it there is much that is also sub-animal and merely vital, much that acts by an instinct and impulse of which the constituting consciousness is withdrawn behind the surface. Below this sub-animal being, there is at a further depth the subvital. When we advance in that ultra-normal self-knowledge and experience which Yoga brings with it, we become aware that the body too has a consciousness of its own; it has habits, impulses, instincts, an inert yet effective will which differs from that of the rest of our being and can resist it and condition its effectiveness. Much of the struggle in our being is due to this composite existence and the interaction of these varied and heterogeneous planes on each other. For man here is the result of an evolution and contains in himself the whole of that evolution up from the merely physical and subvital conscious being to the mental creature which at the top he is.

But this evolution is really a manifestation and just as we have in us these subnormal selves and subhuman planes, so are there in us above our mental being supernormal and superhuman planes. There Chit as the universal conscious-stuff of existence takes other poises, moves out in other modes, on other principles and by other faculties of action. There is above the mind, as the old Vedic sages discovered, a Truth-plane, a plane of self-luminous, self-effective Idea, which can be turned in light and force upon our mind, reason, sentiments, impulses, sensations and use and control them in the sense of the real Truth of things just as we turn our mental reason and will upon our sense-experience and animal nature to use and control them in the sense of our rational and moral perceptions. There there is no seeking, but rather natural possession; no conflict or separation between will and reason, instinct and impulse, desire and experience, idea and reality, but all are in harmony, concomitant, mutually effective, unified in their origin, in their development and in their effectuation. But beyond this plane and attainable through it are others in which the very Chit itself becomes revealed, Chit the elemental origin and primal completeness of all this varied consciousness which is here used for various formation and experience. There will and knowledge and sensation and all the rest of our faculties, powers, modes of experience are not merely harmonious, concomitant, unified, but are one being of consciousness and power of consciousness. It is this Chit which modifies itself so as to become on the Truth-plane the supermind, on the mental plane the mental reason, will, emotion, sensation, on the lower planes the vital or physical instincts, impulses, habits of an obscure force not in superficially conscious possession of itself. All is Chit because all is Sat; all is various movement of the original Consciousness because all is various movement of the original Being.

When we find, see or know Chit, we find also that its essence is Ananda or delight of self-existence. To possess self is to possess self-bliss; not to possess self is to be in more or less obscure search of the delight of existence. Chit eternally possesses its self-bliss; and since Chit is the universal conscious-stuff of being, conscious universal being is also in possession of conscious self-bliss, master of the universal delight of existence. The Divine whether it manifests itself in All-Quality or in No-Quality, in Personality or Impersonality, in the One absorbing the Many or in the One manifesting its essential multiplicity, is always in possession of self-bliss and all-bliss because it is always Sachchidananda. For us also to know and possess our true Self in the essential and the universal is to discover the essential and the universal delight of existence, self-bliss and all-bliss. For the universal is only the pouring out of the essential existence, consciousness and delight; and wherever and in whatever form that manifests as existence, there the essential consciousness must be and therefore there must be an essential delight.

The individual soul does not possess this true nature of itself or realise this true nature of its experience, because it separates itself both from the essential and the universal and identifies itself with the separate accidents, with the unessential form and mode and with the separate aspect and vehicle. Thus it takes its mind, body, life-stream for its essential self. It tries to assert these for their own sake against the universal, against that of which the universal is the manifestation. It is right in trying to assert and fulfil itself in the universal for the sake of something greater and beyond, but wrong in attempting to do so against the universal and in obedience to a fragmentary aspect of the universal. This fragmentary aspect or rather collection of fragmentary experiences it combines around an artificial centre of mental experience, the mental ego, and calls that itself and it serves this ego and lives for its sake instead of living for the sake of that something greater and beyond of which all aspects, even the widest and most general are partial manifestations. This is the living in the false and not the true self; this is living for the sake of and in obedience to the ego and not for the sake of and in obedience to the Divine. The question how this fall has come about and for what purpose it has been done, belongs to the domain of Sankhya rather than of Yoga. We have to seize on the practical fact that to such self-division is due the self-limitation by which we have become unable to possess the true nature of being and experience and are therefore in our mind, life and body subject to ignorance, incapacity and suffering. Non-possession of unity is the root cause; to recover unity is the sovereign means, unity with the universal and with that which the universal is here to express. We have to realise the true self of ourselves and of all; and to realise the true self is to realise Sachchidananda.

---

1. *tattvajñāna.*

# THE DIFFICULTIES OF THE MENTAL BEING

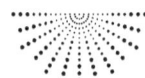

WE HAVE come to this stage in our development of the path of Knowledge that we began by affirming the realisation of our pure self, pure existence above the terms of mind, life and body, as the first object of this Yoga, but we now affirm that this is not sufficient and that we must also realise the Self or Brahman in its essential modes and primarily in its triune reality as Sachchidananda. Not only pure existence, but pure consciousness and pure bliss of its being and consciousness are the reality of the Self and the essence of Brahman.

Further, there are two kinds of realisation of Self or Sachchidananda. One is that of the silent passive quietistic, self-absorbed, self-sufficient existence, consciousness and delight, one, impersonal, without play of qualities, turned away from the infinite phenomenon of the universe or viewing it with indifference and without participation. The other is that of the same existence, consciousness, delight sovereign, free, lord of things, acting out of an inalienable calm, pouring itself out in infinite action and quality out of an eternal self-concentration, the one supreme Person holding in himself all this play of personality in a vast equal impersonality, possessing the infinite phenomenon of the universe without attachment but without any inseparable aloofness, with a divine mastery and an innumerable radiation of his eternal luminous self-delight—as a manifestation which he holds, but by which he is not held, which he governs freely and by which therefore he is not bound. This is not the personal God of the religious or the qualified Brahman of the philosophers, but that in which personal and impersonal, quality and non-quality are reconciled. It is the Transcendent possessing them both in His being and employing them both as modes for His manifestation. This then is the object of realisation for the sadhaka of the integral Yoga.

We see at once that from this point of view the realisation of the pure quiescent self which we gain by withdrawing from mind, life and body, is for us only the acquisition of the necessary basis for this greater realisation. Therefore that process is not sufficient for our Yoga; something else is needed more embracingly positive. As we drew back from all that constitutes our apparent self and the phenomenon of the universe in which it dwells to the self-existent, self-conscious Brahman, so we must now repossess our mind, life and body with the all-embracing self-existence, self-consciousness and self-delight of the Brahman. We must not only have the possession of a pure self-existence independent of the world-play, but possess all existence as our own; not only know ourselves as an infinite unegoistic consciousness beyond all change in Time and Space, but become one with all the outpouring of consciousness and its creative force in Time and Space; not only be capable of a fathomless peace and quiescence, but also of a free and an infinite delight in universal things. For that and not only pure calm is Sachchidananda, is the Brahman.

If it were easily possible to elevate ourselves to the supramental plane and, dwelling securely there, realise world and being, consciousness and action, outgoing and incoming of conscious experience by the power and in the manner of the divine supramental faculties, this realisation would offer no essential difficulties. But man is a mental and not yet a supramental being. It is by the mind therefore that he has to aim at knowledge and realise his being, with whatever help he can get from the supramental planes. This character of our actually realised being and therefore of our Yoga imposes on us certain limitations and primary difficulties which can only be overcome by divine help or an arduous practice, and in reality only by the combination of both these aids. These difficulties in the way of the integral knowledge, the integral realisation, the integral becoming we have to state succinctly before we can proceed farther.

Realised mental being and realised spiritual being are really two different planes in the arrangement of our existence, the one superior and divine, the other inferior and human. To the former belong infinite being, infinite consciousness and will, infinite bliss and the infinite comprehensive and self-effective knowledge of supermind, four divine principles; to the latter belong mental being, vital being, physical being, three human principles. In their apparent nature the two are opposed; each is the reverse of the other. The divine is infinite and immortal being; the human is life limited in time and scope and form, life that is death attempting to become life that is immortality. The divine is infinite consciousness transcending and embracing all that it manifests within it; the human is consciousness rescued from a sleep of inconscience, subjected to the means it uses, limited by body and ego and attempting to find its relation to other consciousnesses, bodies, egos positively by various means of uniting contact and sympathy, negatively by various means of hostile contact and antipathy. The divine is inalienable self-bliss and inviolable all-bliss; the human is sensation of mind and body seeking for delight, but finding only pleasure, indifference and pain. The divine is supramental knowledge comprehending all and supramental will effecting all; the human is ignorance reaching out to knowledge by the comprehension of things in parts and parcels which it has to join clumsily together, and it is incapacity attempting to acquire force and will through a gradual extension of power corresponding to its gradual extension of knowledge; and this extension it can only bring about by a partial and parcelled exercise of will corresponding to the partial and parcelled method of its knowledge. The divine founds itself upon unity and is master of the transcendences and totalities of things; the human founds itself on separated multiplicity and is the subject even when the master of their division and fragmentations and their difficult solderings and unifyings. Between the two there are for the human being a veil and a lid which prevent the human not only from attaining but even from knowing the divine.

When, therefore, the mental being seeks to know the divine, to realise it, to become it, it has first to lift this lid, to put by this veil. But when it succeeds in that difficult endeavour, it sees the divine as something superior to it, distant, high, conceptually, vitally, even physically above it, to which it looks up from its own humble station and to which it has, if at all that be possible, to rise, or if it be not possible, to call that down to itself, to be subject to it and to adore. It sees the divine as a superior plane of being, and then it regards it as a supreme state of existence, a heaven or a Sat or a Nirvana according to the nature of its own conception or realisation. Or it sees it as a supreme Being other than itself or at least other than its own present self, and then it calls it God under one name or another, and views it as personal or impersonal, qualitied or without qualities, silent and indifferent Power or active Lord and Helper, again according to its own conception or realisation, its vision or understanding of some side or some aspect of that Being. Or it sees it as a supreme Reality of which its own imperfect being is a reflection or from which it has become detached, and then it calls it Self or Brahman and qualifies it variously, always according to its own conception or realisation,—Existence, Non-Existence, Tao, Nihil, Force, Unknowable.

If then we seek mentally to realise Sachchidananda, there is likely to be this first difficulty that we shall see it as something above, beyond, around even in a sense, but with a gulf between that being and our being, an unbridged or even an unbridgeable chasm. There is this infinite existence; but it is quite other than the mental being who becomes aware of it, and we cannot either raise ourselves to it and become it or bring it down to ourselves so that our own experience of our being and world-being shall be that of its blissful infinity. There is this great, boundless, unconditioned consciousness and force; but our consciousness and force stands apart from it, even if within it, limited, petty, discouraged, disgusted with itself and the world, but unable to participate in that higher thing which it has seen. There is this immeasurable and unstained bliss; but our own being remains the sport of a lower Nature of pleasure and pain and dull neutral sensation incapable of its divine delight. There is this perfect Knowledge and Will; but our own remains always the mental deformed knowledge and limping will incapable of sharing in or even being in tune with that nature of Godhead. Or else so long as we live purely in an ecstatic contemplation of that vision, we are delivered from ourselves; but the moment we again turn our consciousness upon our own being, we fall away from it and it disappears or becomes remote and intangible. The Divinity leaves us; the Vision vanishes; we are back again in the pettiness of our mortal existence.

Somehow this chasm has to be bridged. And here there are two possibilities for the mental being. One possibility is for it to rise by a great, prolonged, concentrated, all-forgetting effort out of itself into the Supreme. But in this effort the mind has to leave its own consciousness, to disappear into another and temporarily or permanently lose itself, if not quite abolish. It has to go into the trance of Samadhi. For this reason the Raja and other systems of Yoga give a supreme importance to the state of Samadhi or Yogic trance in which the mind withdraws not only from its ordinary interests and preoccupations, but first from all consciousness of outward act and sense and being and then from all consciousness of inward mental activities. In this its inward-gathered state the mental being may have different kinds of realisation of the Supreme in itself or in various aspects or on various levels, but the ideal is to get rid of mind altogether and, going beyond mental realisation, to enter into the absolute trance in which all sign of mind or lower existence ceases. But this is a state of consciousness to which few can attain and from which not all can return.

It is obvious, since mind-consciousness is the sole waking state possessed by mental being, that it cannot ordinarily quite enter into another without leaving behind completely both all our waking existence and all our inward mind. This is the necessity of the Yogic trance. But one cannot continually remain in this trance; or, even if one could persist in it for an indefinitely long period, it is always likely to be broken in upon by any strong or persistent call on the bodily life. And when one returns to the mental consciousness, one is back again in the lower being. Therefore it has been said that complete liberation from the human birth, complete ascension from the life of the mental being is impossible until the body and the bodily life are finally cast off. The ideal upheld before the Yogin who follows this method is to renounce all desire and every least velleity of the human life, of the mental existence, to detach himself utterly from the world and, entering more and more frequently and more and more deeply into the most concentrated state of Samadhi, finally to leave the body while in that utter in-gathering of the being so that it may depart into the supreme Existence. It is also by reason of this apparent incompatibility of mind and Spirit that so many religions and systems are led to condemn the world and look forward only to a heaven beyond or else a void Nirvana or supreme featureless self-existence in the Supreme.

But what under these circumstances is the human mind which seeks the divine to do with its waking moments? For if these are subject to all the disabilities of mortal mentality, if they are open to the attacks of grief, fear, anger, passion, hunger, greed, desire, it is irrational to suppose that by the mere concentration of the mental being in the Yogic trance at the moment of putting off the body, the soul can pass away without return into the supreme existence. For the man's normal consciousness is still subject to what the Buddhists call the chain or the stream of Karma; it is still creating energies which must continue and have their effect in a continued life of the mental being which is creating them. Or, to take another point of view, consciousness being the determining fact and not the bodily existence which is only a result, the man still belongs normally to the status of human, or at least mental activity and his cannot be abrogated by the fact of passing out of the physical body; to get rid of mortal body is not to get rid of mortal mind. Nor is it sufficient to have a dominant disgust of the world or an anti-vital indifference or aversion to the material existence; for this too belongs to the lower mental status and activity. The highest teaching is that even the desire for liberation with all its mental concomitants must be surpassed before the soul can be entirely free. Therefore not only must the mind be able to rise in abnormal states out of itself into a higher consciousness, but its waking mentality also must be entirely spiritualised.

This brings into the field the second possibility open to the mental being; for if its first possibility is to rise out of itself into a divine supramental plane of being, the other is to call down the divine into itself so that its mentality shall be changed into an image of the divine, shall be divinised or spiritualised. This may be done and primarily must be done by the mind's power of reflecting that which it knows, relates to its own consciousness, contemplates. For the mind is really a reflector and a medium and none of its activities originate in themselves, none exist *per se*. Ordinarily, the mind reflects the status of mortal nature and the activities of the Force which works under the conditions of the material universe. But if it becomes clear, passive, pure by the renunciation of these activities and of the characteristic ideas and outlook of mental nature, then as in a clear mirror or like the sky in clear water which is without ripple and unruffled by winds, the divine is reflected. The mind still does not entirely possess the divine or become divine, but is possessed by it or by a luminous reflection of it so long as it remains in this pure passivity. If it becomes active, it falls back into the disturbance of the mortal nature and reflects that and no longer the divine. For this reason an absolute quietism and a cessation first of all outer action and then of all inner movement is the ideal ordinarily proposed; here too, for the follower of the path of knowledge, there must be a sort of waking Samadhi. Whatever action is unavoidable, must be a purely superficial working of the organs of perception and motor action in which the quiescent mind takes eventually no part and from which it seeks no result or profit.

But this is insufficient for the integral Yoga. There must be a positive transformation and not merely a negative quiescence of the waking mentality. The transformation is possible because, although the divine planes are above the mental consciousness and to enter actually into them we have ordinarily to lose the mental in Samadhi, yet there are in the mental being divine planes superior to our normal mentality which reproduce the conditions of the divine plane proper, although modified by the conditions, dominant here, of mentality. All that belongs to the experience of the divine plane can there be seized, but in the mental way and in a mental form. To these planes of divine mentality it is possible for the developed human being to arise in the waking state; or it is possible for him to derive from them a stream of influences and experiences which shall eventually open to them and transform into their nature his whole waking existence. These higher mental states are the immediate sources, the large actual instruments, the inner stations[1] of his perfection.

But in arriving to these planes or deriving from them the limitations of our mentality pursue us. In the first place the mind is an inveterate divider of the indivisible and its whole nature is to dwell on one thing at a time to the exclusion of others or to stress it to the subordination of others. Thus in approaching Sachchidananda it will dwell on its aspect of the pure existence, Sat, and consciousness and bliss are compelled then to lose themselves or remain quiescent in the experience of pure, infinite being which leads to the realisation of the quietistic Monist. Or it will dwell on the aspect of consciousness, Chit, and existence and bliss become then dependent on the experience of an infinite transcendent Power and Conscious-Force, which leads to the realisation of the Tantric worshipper of Energy. Or it will dwell on the aspect of delight, Ananda, and existence and consciousness then seem to disappear into a bliss without basis of self-possessing awareness or constituent being, which leads to the realisation of the Buddhistic seeker of Nirvana. Or it will dwell on some aspect of Sachchidananda which comes to the mind from the supramental Knowledge, Will or Love, and then the infinite impersonal aspect of Sachchidananda is almost or quite lost in the experience of the Deity which leads to the realisations of the various religions and to the possession of some supernal world or divine status of the human soul in relation to God. And for those whose object is to depart anywhither from cosmic existence, this is enough, since they are able by the mind's immergence into or seizure upon any one of these principles or aspects to effect through status in the divine planes of their mentality or the possession by them of their waking state this desired transit.

But the sadhaka of the integral Yoga has to harmonise all so that they may become a plenary and equal unity of the full realisation of Sachchidananda. Here the last difficulty of mind meets him, its inability to hold at once the unity and the multiplicity. It is not altogether difficult to arrive at and dwell in a pure infinite or even, at the same time, a perfect global experience of the Existence which is Consciousness which is Delight. The mind may even extend its experience of this Unity to the multiplicity so as to perceive it immanent in the universe and in each object, force, movement in the universe or at the same time to be aware of this Existence-Consciousness-Bliss containing the universe and enveloping all its objects and originating all its movements. It is difficult indeed for it to unite and harmonise rightly all these experiences; but still it can possess Sachchidananda at once in himself and immanent in all and the continent of all. But with this to unite the final experience of all this as Sachchidananda and possess objects, movements, forces, forms as no other than He, is the great difficulty for mind. Separately any of these things may be done; the mind may go from one to the other, rejecting one as it arrives at another and calling this the lower or that the higher existence. But to unify without losing, to integralise without rejecting is its supreme difficulty.

---

1. Called in the Veda variously seats, houses, placings or statuses, footings, earths, dwelling-places, *sadas, gṛha* or *kṣaya, dhāma, padam, bhūmi, kṣiti.*

# THE PASSIVE AND THE ACTIVE BRAHMAN

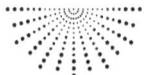

THE DIFFICULTY which the mental being experiences in arriving at an integral realisation of true being and world-being may be met by following one or other of two different lines of his self-development. He may evolve himself from plane to plane of his own being and embrace on each successively his oneness with the world and with Sachchidananda realised as the Purusha and Prakriti, Conscious-Soul and Nature-Soul of that plane, taking into himself the action of the lower grades of being as he ascends. He may, that is to say, work out by a sort of inclusive process of self-enlargement and transformation the evolution of the material into the divine or spiritual man. This seems to have been the method of the most ancient sages of which we get some glimpse in the Rig Veda and some of the Upanishads.[1] He may, on the other hand, aim straight at the realisation of pure self-existence on the highest plane of mental being and from that secure basis realise spiritually under the conditions of his mentality the process by which the self-existent becomes all existences, but without that descent into the self-divided egoistic consciousness which is a circumstance of evolution in the Ignorance. Thus identified with Sachchidananda in the universal self-existence as the spiritualised mental being, he may then ascend beyond to the supramental plane of the pure spiritual existence. It is the latter method the stages of which we may now attempt to trace for the seeker by the path of knowledge.

When the sadhaka has followed the discipline of withdrawal from the various identifications of the self with the ego, the mind, the life, the body, he has arrived at realisation by knowledge of a pure, still, self-aware existence, one, undivided, peaceful, inactive, undisturbed by the action of the world. The only relation that this Self seems to have with the world is that of a disinterested Witness not at all involved in or affected or even touched by any of its activities. If this state of consciousness is pushed farther one becomes aware of a self even more remote from world-existence; all that is in the world is in a sense in that Self and yet at the same time extraneous to its consciousness, non-existent in its existence, existing only in a sort of unreal mind,—a dream therefore, an illusion. This aloof and transcendent Real Existence may be realised as an utter Self of one's own being; or the very idea of a self and of one's own being may be swallowed up in it, so that it is only for the mind an unknowable That, unknowable to the mental consciousness and without any possible kind of actual connection or commerce with world-existence. It can even be realised by the mental being as a Nihil, Non-Existence or Void, but a Void of all that is in the world, a Non-existence of all that is in the world and yet the only Reality. To proceed farther towards that Transcendence by concentration of one's own being upon it is to lose mental existence and world-existence altogether and cast oneself into the Unknowable.

The integral Yoga of knowledge demands instead a divine return upon world-existence and its first step must be to realise the Self as the All, *sarvaṁ brahma*. First, concentrating on the Self-existent, we have to realise all of which the mind and senses are aware as a figure of things existing in this pure Self that we now are to our own consciousness. This vision of the pure self translates itself to the mind-sense and the mind-perception as an infinite Reality in which all exists merely as name and form, not precisely unreal, not a hallucination or a dream, but still only a creation of the consciousness, perceptual and subtly sensible rather than substantial. In this poise of the consciousness all seems to be, if not a dream, yet very much like a representation or puppet-show taking place in the calm, motionless, peaceful, indifferent Self. Our own phenomenal existence is part of this conceptual movement, a mechanical form of mind and body among other forms, ourselves a name of being among other names, automatically mobile in this Self with its all-encompassing, still self-awareness. The active consciousness of the world is not present in this state to our realisation, because thought has been stilled in us and therefore our own consciousness is perfectly still and inactive,—whatever we do, seems to be purely mechanical, not attended with any conscious origination by our active will and knowledge. Or if thought occurs, that also happens mechanically like the rest, like the movement of our body, moved by the unseen springs of Nature as in the plant and element and not by any active will of our self-existence. For this Self is the immobile and does not originate or take part in the action which it allows. This Self is the All in the sense only of being the infinite One who is immutably and contains all names and forms.

The basis of this status of consciousness is the mind's exclusive realisation of pure self-existence in which consciousness is at rest, inactive, widely concentrated in pure self-awareness of being, not active and originative of any kind of becoming. Its aspect of knowledge is at rest in the awareness of undifferentiated identity; its aspect of force and will is at rest in the awareness of unmodifiable immutability. And yet it is aware of names and forms, it is aware of movement; but this movement does not seem to proceed from the Self, but to go on by some inherent power of its own and only to be reflected in the Self. In other words, the mental being has put away from himself by exclusive concentration the dynamic aspect of consciousness, has taken refuge in the static and built a wall of non-communication between the two; between the passive and the active Brahman a gulf has been created and they stand on either side of it, the one visible to the other but with no contact, no touch of sympathy, no sense of unity between them. Therefore to the passive Self all conscious being seems to be passive in its nature, all activity seems to be non-conscious in itself and mechanical (*jaḍa*) in its movement. The realisation of this status is the basis of the ancient Sankhya philosophy which taught that the Purusha or Conscious-Soul is a passive, inactive, immutable entity, Prakriti or the Nature-Soul including even the mind and the understanding active, mutable, mechanical, but reflected in the Purusha which identifies itself with what is reflected in it and lends to it its own light of consciousness. When the Purusha learns not to identify himself, then Prakriti begins to fall away from its impulse of movement and returns towards equilibrium and rest. The Vedantic view of the same status led to the philosophy of the inactive Self or Brahman as the one reality and of all the rest as name and form imposed on it by a false activity of mental illusion which has to be removed by right knowledge of the immutable Self and refusal of the imposition.[2] The two views really differ only in their language and their view-point; substantially, they are the same intellectual generalisation from the same spiritual experience.

If we rest here, there are only two possible attitudes towards the world. Either we must remain as mere inactive witnesses of the world-play or act in it mechanically without any participation of the conscious self and by mere play of the organs of sense and motor-action.[3] In the former choice what we do is to approach as completely as possible to the inactivity of the passive and silent Brahman. We have stilled our mind and silenced the activity of the thought and the disturbances of the heart, we have arrived at an entire inner peace and indifference; we attempt now to still the mechanical action of the life and body, to reduce it to the most meagre minimum possible so that it may eventually cease entirely and for ever. This, the final aim of the ascetic Yoga which refuses life, is evidently not our aim. By the alternative choice we can have an activity perfect enough in outward appearance along with an entire inner passivity, peace, mental silence, indifference and cessation of the emotions, absence of choice in the will.

To the ordinary mind this does not seem possible. As, emotionally, it cannot conceive of activity without desire and emotional preference, so intellectually it cannot conceive of activity without thought-conception, conscious motive and energising of the will. But, as a matter of fact, we see that a large part of our own action as well as the whole activity of inanimate and merely animate life is done by a mechanical impulse and movement in which these elements are not, openly at least, at work. It may be said that this is only possible of the purely physical and vital activity and not of those movements which ordinarily depend upon the functioning of the conceptual and volitional mind, such as speech, writing and all the intelligent action of human life. But this again is not true, as we find when we are able to go behind the habitual and normal process of our mental nature. It has been found by recent psychological experiment that all these operations can be effected without any conscious origination in the thought and will of the apparent actor; his organs of sense and action, including the speech, become passive instruments for a thought and will other than his.

Certainly, behind all intelligent action there must be an intelligent will, but it need not be the intelligence or the will of the conscious mind in the actor. In the psychological phenomena of which I have spoken, it is obviously in some of them the will and intelligence of other human beings that uses the organs, in others it is doubtful whether it is an influence or actuation by other beings or the emergence of a subconscious, subliminal mind or a mixed combination of both these agencies. But in this Yogic status of action by the mere organs, *kevalair indriyair*, it is the universal intelligence and will of Nature itself working from centres superconscious and subconscious as it acts in the mechanically purposeful energies of plant-life or of the inanimate material form, but here with a living instrument who is the conscious witness of the action and instrumentation. It is a remarkable fact that the speech, writing and intelligent actions of such a state may convey a perfect force of thought, luminous, faultless, logical, inspired, perfectly adapting means to ends, far beyond what the man himself could have done in his old normal poise of mind and will and capacity, yet all the time he himself perceives but does not conceive the thought that comes to him, observes in its works but does not appropriate or use the will that acts through him, witnesses but does not claim as his own the powers which play upon the world through him as through a passive channel. But this phenomenon is not really abnormal or contrary to the general law of things. For do we not see a perfect working of the secret universal Will and Intelligence in the apparently brute (*jaḍa*) action of material Nature? And it is precisely this universal Will and Intelligence which thus acts through the calm, indifferent and inwardly silent Yogin who offers no obstacle of limited and ignorant personal will and intelligence to its operations. He dwells in the silent Self; he allows the active Brahman to work through his natural instruments, accepting impartially, without participation, the formations of its universal force and knowledge.

This status of an inner passivity and an outer action independent of each other is a state of entire spiritual freedom. The Yogin, as the Gita says, even in acting does no actions, for it is not he, but universal Nature directed by the Lord of Nature which is at work. He is not bound by his works, nor do they leave any after effects or consequences in his mind, nor cling to or leave any mark on his soul;[4] they vanish and are dissolved[5] by their very execution and leave the immutable self unaffected and the soul unmodified. Therefore this would seem to be the poise the uplifted soul ought to take, if it has still to preserve any relations with human action in the world-existence, an unalterable silence, tranquillity, passivity within, an action without regulated by the universal Will and Wisdom which works, as the Gita says, without being involved in, bound by or ignorantly attached to its works. And certainly this poise of a perfect activity founded upon a perfect inner passivity is that which the Yogin has to possess, as we have seen in the Yoga of Works. But here in this status of self-knowledge at which we have arrived, there is an evident absence of integrality; for there is still a gulf, an unrealised unity or a cleft of consciousness between the passive and the active Brahman. We have still to possess consciously the active Brahman without losing the possession of the silent Self. We have to preserve the inner silence, tranquillity, passivity as a foundation; but in place of an aloof indifference to the works of the active Brahman we have to arrive at an equal and impartial delight in them; in place of a refusal to participate lest our freedom and peace be lost we have to arrive at a conscious possession of the active Brahman whose joy of existence does not abrogate His peace, nor His lordship of all workings impair His calm freedom in the midst of His works.

The difficulty is created by the exclusive concentration of the mental being on its plane of pure existence in which consciousness is at rest in passivity and delight of existence at rest in peace of existence. It has to embrace also its plane of conscious force of existence in which consciousness is active as power and will and delight is active as joy of existence. Here the difficulty is that mind is likely to precipitate itself into the consciousness of Force instead of possessing it. The extreme mental state of precipitation into Nature is that of the ordinary man who takes his bodily and vital activity and the mind-movements dependent on them for his whole real existence and regards all passivity of the soul as a departure from existence and an approach towards nullity. He lives in the superficies of the active Brahman and while to the silent soul exclusively concentrated in the passive self all activities are mere name and form, to him they are the only reality and it is the Self that is merely a name. In one the passive Brahman stands aloof from the active and does not share in its consciousness; in the other the active Brahman stands aloof from the passive and does not share in its consciousness nor wholly possess its own. Each is to the other in these exclusivenesses an inertia of status or an inertia of mechanically active non-possession of self if not altogether an unreality. But the sadhaka who has once seen firmly the essence of things and tasted thoroughly the peace of the silent Self, is not likely to be content with any state which involves loss of self-knowledge or a sacrifice of the peace of the soul. He will not precipitate himself back into the mere individual movement of mind and life and body with all its ignorance and straining and disturbance. Whatever new status he may acquire, will only satisfy him if it is founded upon and includes that which he has already found to be indispensable to real self-knowledge, self-delight and self-possession.

Still there is the likelihood of a partial, superficial and temporary relapse into the old mental movement when he attempts again to ally himself to the activity of the world. To prevent this relapse or to cure it when it arrives, he has to hold fast to the truth of Sachchidananda and extend his realisation of the infinite One into the movement of the infinite multiplicity. He has to concentrate on and realise the one Brahman in all things as conscious force of being as well as pure awareness of conscious being. The Self as the All, not only in the unique essence of things, but in the manifold form of things, not only as containing all in a transcendent consciousness, but as becoming all by a constituting consciousness, this is the next step towards his true possession of existence. In proportion as this realisation is accomplished, the status of consciousness as well as the mental view proper to it will change. Instead of an immutable Self containing name and form, containing without sharing in them the mutations of Nature, there will be the consciousness of the Self immutable in essence, unalterable in its fundamental poise but constituting and becoming in its experience all these existences which the mind distinguishes as name and form. All formations of mind and body will be not merely figures reflected in the Purusha, but real forms of which Brahman, Self, conscious Being is the substance and, as it were, the material of their formation. The name attaching to the form will be not a mere conception of the mind answering to no real existence bearing the name, but there will be behind it a true power of conscious being, a true self-experience of the Brahman answering to something that it contained potential but unmanifest in its silence. And yet in all its mutations it will be realised as one, free and above them. The realisation of a sole Reality suffering the imposition of names and forms will give place to that of eternal Being throwing itself out into infinite becoming. All existences will be to the consciousness of the Yogin soul-forms and not merely idea-forms of the Self, of himself, one with him, contained in his universal existence. All the soul-life, mental, vital, bodily existence of all that exists will be to him one indivisible movement and activity of the Being who is the same forever. The Self will be realised as the all in its double aspect of immutable status and mutable activity and it is this that will be seen as the comprehensive truth of our existence.

1. Notably, the Taittiriya Upanishad.
2. *adhyāropa*.
3. *kevalair indriyair*. Gita.
4. *na karma lipyate nare*. Isha Upanishad.
5. *pravilīyante karmāṇi* Gita.

# THE COSMIC CONSCIOUSNESS

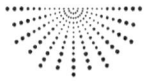

TO REALISE and unite oneself with the active Brahman is to exchange, perfectly or imperfectly according as the union is partial or complete, the individual for the cosmic consciousness. The ordinary existence of man is not only an individual but an egoistic consciousness; it is, that is to say, the individual soul or Jivatman identifying himself with the nodus of his mental, vital, physical experiences in the movement of universal Nature, that is to say, with his mind-created ego, and, less intimately, with the mind, life, body which receive the experiences. Less intimately, because of these he can say "my mind, life, body," he can regard them as himself, yet partly as not himself and something rather which he possesses and uses, but of the ego he says, "It is I." By detaching himself from all identification with mind, life and body, he can get back from his ego to the consciousness of the true Individual, the Jivatman, who is the real possessor of mind, life and body. Looking back from this Individual to that of which it is the representative and conscious figure, he can get back to the transcendent consciousness of pure Self, absolute Existence or absolute Non-being, three poises of the same eternal Reality. But between the movement of universal Nature and this transcendent Existence, possessor of the one and cosmic self of the other, is the cosmic consciousness, the universal Purusha of whom all Nature is the Prakriti or active conscious Force. We can arrive at that, become that whether by breaking the walls of the ego laterally, as it were, and identifying oneself with all existences in the One, or else from above by realising the pure Self or absolute Existence in its outgoing, immanent, all-embracing, all-constituting self-knowledge and self-creative power.

The immanent, silent Self in all is the foundation of this cosmic consciousness for the experience of the mental being. It is the Witness pure and omnipresent who as the silent Conscious Soul of the cosmos regards all the activity of the universe; it is Sachchidananda for whose delight universal Nature displays the eternal procession of her works. We are aware of an un-wounded Delight, a pure and perfect Presence, an infinite and self-contained Power present in ourselves and all things, not divided by their divisions, not affected by the stress and struggle of the cosmic manifestation; it is within it all, but it is superior to it all. Because of that all this exists, but that does not exist because of all this; it is too great to be limited by the movement in Time and Space which it inhabits and supports. This foundation enables us to possess in the security of the divine existence the whole universe within our own being. We are no longer limited and shut in by what we inhabit, but like the Divine contain in ourselves all that for the purpose of the movement of Nature we consent to inhabit. We are not mind or life or body, but the informing and sustaining Soul, silent, peaceful, eternal, which possesses them; and since we find this Soul everywhere sustaining and informing and possessing all lives and minds and bodies, we cease to regard it as a separate and individual being in our own. In it all this moves and acts; within all this it is stable and immutable. Having this, we possess our eternal self-existence at rest in its eternal consciousness and bliss.

Next we have to realise this silent Self as the Lord of all the action of universal Nature; we have to see that it is this same Self-existent who is displayed in the creative force of His eternal consciousness. All this action is only His power and knowledge and self-delight going abroad in His infinite being to do the works of His eternal wisdom and will. We shall realise the Divine, the eternal Self of all, first, as the source of all action and inaction, of all knowledge and ignorance, of all delight and suffering, of all good and evil, perfection and imperfection, of all force and form, of all the outgoing of Nature from the eternal divine Principle and of all the return of Nature towards the Divine. We shall realise it next as itself going abroad in its Power and Knowledge,—for the Power and Knowledge are itself,—not only the source of their works, but the creator and doer of their works, one in all existences; for the many souls of the universal manifestation are only faces of the one Divine, the many minds, lives, bodies are only His masks and disguises. We perceive each being to be the universal Narayana presenting to us many faces; we lose ourselves in that universality and perceive our own mind, life and body as only one presentation of the Self, while all whom we formerly conceived of as others, are now to our consciousness our self in other minds, lives and bodies. All force and idea and event and figure of things in the universe are only manifest degrees of this Self, values of the Divine in His eternal self-figuration. Thus viewing things and beings we may see them first as if they were parts and parcels of His divided being;[1] but the realisation and the knowledge are not complete unless we go beyond this idea of quality and space and division by which there comes the experience of less and more, large and small, part and whole, and see the whole Infinite everywhere; we must see the universe and each thing in the universe as in its existence and secret consciousness and power and delight the indivisible Divine in its entirety, however much the figure it makes to our minds may appear only as a partial manifestation. When we possess thus the Divine as at once the silent and surpassing Witness and the active Lord and all-constituting Being without making any division between these aspects, we possess the whole cosmic Divine, embrace all of the universal Self and Reality, are awake to the cosmic consciousness.

What will be the relation of our individual existence to this cosmic consciousness to which we have attained? For since we have still a mind and body and human life, our individual existence persists even though our separate individual consciousness has been transcended. It is quite possible to realise the cosmic consciousness without becoming that; we can see it, that is to say, with the soul, feel it and dwell in it; we can even be united with it without becoming wholly one with it; in a word, we may preserve the individual consciousness of the Jivatman within the cosmic consciousness of the universal Self. We may preserve a yet greater distinctness between the two and enjoy the relations between them; we may remain, in a way, entirely the individual self while participating in the bliss and infinity of the universal Self. Or we may possess them both as a greater and lesser self, one we feel pouring itself out in the universal play of the divine consciousness and force, the other in the action of the same universal Being through our individual soul-centre or soul-form for the purposes of an individual play of mind, life and body. But the summit of this cosmic realisation by knowledge is always the power to dissolve the personality in universal being, to merge the individual in the cosmic consciousness, to liberate even the soul-form into the unity and universality of the Spirit. This is the *laya*, dissolution, or *mokṣa*, liberation, at which the Yoga of Knowledge aims. This may extend itself, as in the traditional Yoga, to the dissolution of mind, life and body itself into the silent Self or absolute Existence; but the essence of the liberation is the merging of the individual in the Infinite. When the Yogin no longer feels himself to be a consciousness situated in the body or limited by the mind, but has lost the sense of division in the boundlessness of an infinite consciousness, that which he set out to do is accomplished. Afterwards the retaining or non-retaining of the human life is a circumstance of no essential importance, for it is always the formless One who acts through its many forms of the mind and life and body and each soul is only one of the stations from which it chooses to watch and receive and actuate its own play.

That into which we merge ourselves in the cosmic consciousness is Sachchidananda. It is one eternal Existence that we then are, one eternal Consciousness which sees its own works in us and others, one eternal Will or Force of that Consciousness which displays itself in infinite workings, one eternal Delight which has the joy of itself and all its workings. It is itself stable, immutable, timeless, spaceless, supreme and it is still itself in the infinity of its workings, not changed by their variations, not broken up by their multiplicity, not increased or diminished by their ebbings and flowings in the seas of Time and Space, not confused by their apparent contrarieties or limited by their divinely-willed limitations. Sachchidananda is the unity of the many-sidedness of manifested things, Sachchidananda is the eternal harmony of all their variations and oppositions, Sachchidananda is the infinite perfection which justifies their limitations and is the goal of their imperfections.

So much for the essential relation; but we have to see also the practical results of this internal transformation. It is evident that by dwelling in this cosmic consciousness our whole experience and valuation of everything in the universe will be radically changed. As individual egos we dwell in the Ignorance and judge everything by a broken, partial and personal standard of knowledge; we experience everything according to the capacity of a limited consciousness and force and are therefore unable to give a divine response or set the true value upon any part of cosmic experience. We experience limitation, weakness, incapacity, grief, pain, struggle and its contradictory emotions and we accept these things and their opposites as opposites in an eternal duality and cannot reconcile them in the eternity of an absolute good and happiness. We live by fragments of experience and judge by our fragmentary values each thing and the whole. When we try to arrive at absolute values we only promote some partial view of things to do duty for a totality in the divine workings; we then make believe that our fractions are integers and try to thrust our one-sided view-points into the catholicity of the all-vision of the Divine.

But by entering into the cosmic consciousness we begin to participate in that all-vision and see everything in the values of the Infinite and the One. Limitation itself, ignorance itself change their meaning for us. Ignorance changes into a particularising action of divine knowledge; strength and weakness and incapacity change into a free putting forth and holding back various measures of divine Force; joy and grief, pleasure and pain change into a mastering and a suffering of divine delight; struggle, losing its discords, becomes a balancing of forces and values in the divine harmony. We do not then suffer by the limitations of our mind, life and body; for we no longer live in these, even when we record and accept them, but in the infinity of the Spirit, and these we view in their right value and place and purpose in the manifestation, as degrees of the supreme being, conscious-force and delight of Sachchidananda veiling and manifesting Himself in the cosmos. We cease also to judge other men and things by their outward appearances and are delivered from hostile and contradictory ideas and emotions; for it is the soul that we see, the Divine that we seek and find in every thing and creature, and the rest has only a secondary value to us in a scheme of relations which exist now for us only as self-expressions of the Divine and not as having any absolute value in themselves. So too no event can disturb us, since the distinction of happy and unhappy, beneficent and maleficent happenings loses its force, and all is seen in its divine value and its divine purpose. Thus we arrive at a perfect liberation and an infinite equality. It is this consummation of which the Upanishad speaks when it says "He in whom the self has become all existences, how shall he have delusion, whence shall he have grief who knows entirely[2] and sees in all things oneness."

But this can be only when there is perfection in the cosmic consciousness, and that is difficult for the mental being. The mentality when it arrives at the idea or the realisation of the Spirit, the Divine, tends to break existence into two opposite halves, the lower and the higher existence. It sees on one side the Infinite, the Formless, the One, the Peace and Bliss, the Calm and Silence, the Absolute, the Vast and Pure; on the other it sees the finite, the world of forms, the jarring multiplicity, the strife and suffering and imperfect, unreal good, the tormented activity and futile success, the relative, the limited and vain and vile. To those who make this division and this opposition, complete liberation is only attainable in the peace of the One, in the featurelessness of the Infinite, in the non-becoming of the Absolute which is to them the only real being; to be free all values must be destroyed, all limitations not only transcended but abolished.

They have the liberation of the divine rest, but not the liberty of the divine action; they enjoy the peace of the Transcendent, but not the cosmic bliss of the Transcendent. Their liberty depends upon abstention from the cosmic movement, it cannot dominate and possess cosmic existence itself. But it is also possible for them to realise and participate in the immanent as well as the transcendent peace. Still the division is not cured. The liberty they enjoy is that of the silent unacting Witness, not the liberty of the divine Master-consciousness which possesses all things, delights in all, casts itself into all forms of existence without fear of fall or loss or bondage or stain. All the rights of the Spirit are not yet possessed; there is still a denial, a limitation, a holding back from the entire oneness of all existence. The workings of Mind, Life, Body are viewed from the calm and peace of the spiritual planes of the mental being and are filled with that calm and peace; they are not possessed by and subjected to the law of the all-mastering Spirit.

All this is when the mental being takes its station in its own spiritual planes, in the mental planes of Sat, Chit, Ananda, and casts down their light and delight upon the lower existence. But there is possible the attempt at a kind of cosmic consciousness by dwelling on the lower planes themselves after breaking their limitations laterally, as we have said, and then calling down into them the light and largeness of the higher existence. Not only Spirit is one, but Mind, Life, Matter are one. There is one cosmic Mind, one cosmic life, one cosmic Body. All the attempt of man to arrive at universal sympathy, universal love and the understanding and knowledge of the inner soul of other existences is an attempt to beat thin, breach and eventually break down by the power of the enlarging mind and heart the walls of the ego and arrive nearer to a cosmic oneness. And if we can by the mind and heart get at the touch of the Spirit, receive the powerful inrush of the Divine into this lower humanity and change our nature into a reflection of the divine nature by love, by universal joy, by oneness of mind with all Nature and all beings, we can break down the walls. Even our bodies are not really separate entities and therefore our very physical consciousness is capable of oneness with the physical consciousness of others and of the cosmos. The Yogin is able to feel his body one with all bodies, to be aware of and even to participate in their affections; he can feel constantly the unity of all Matter and be aware of his physical being as only a movement in its movement.[3] Still more is it possible for him to feel constantly and normally the whole sea of the infinite life as his true vital existence and his own life as only a wave of that boundless surge. And more easily yet is it possible for him to unite himself in mind and heart with all existences, be aware of their desires, struggles, joys, sorrows, thoughts, impulses, in a sense as if they were his own, at least as occurring in his larger self hardly less intimately or quite as intimately as the movements of his own heart and mind. This too is a realisation of cosmic consciousness.

It may even seem as if it were the greatest oneness, since it accepts all that we can be sensible of in the mind-created world as our own. Sometimes one sees it spoken of as the highest achievement. Certainly, it is a great realisation and the path to a greater. It is that which the Gita speaks of as the accepting of all existences as if oneself whether in grief or in joy; it is the way of sympathetic oneness and infinite compassion which helps the Buddhist to arrive at his Nirvana. Still there are gradations and degrees. In the first stage the soul is still subject to the reactions of the duality, still subject therefore to the lower Prakriti; it is depressed or hurt by the cosmic suffering, elated by the cosmic joy. We suffer the joys of others, suffer their griefs; and this oneness can be carried even into the body, as in the story of the Indian saint who, seeing a bullock tortured in the field by its cruel owner, cried out with the creature's pain and the weal of the lash was found reproduced on his own flesh. But there must be a oneness with Sachchidananda in his freedom as well as with the subjection of the lower being to the reactions of Prakriti. This is achieved when the soul is free and superior to the cosmic reactions which are then felt only in the life, mind and body and as an inferior movement; the soul understands, accepts the experience, sympathises, but is not overpowered or affected, so that at last even the mind and body learn also to accept without being overpowered or even affected except on their surface. And the consummation of this movement is when the two spheres of existence are no longer divided and the mind, life and body obeying utterly the higher law grow into the spirit's freedom; free from the lower or ignorant response to the cosmic touches, their struggle and their subjection to the duality ceases. This does not mean insensibility to the subjection and struggles and sufferings of others, but it does mean a spiritual supremacy and freedom which enables one to understand perfectly, put the right values on things and heal from above instead of struggling from below. It does not inhibit the divine compassion and helpfulness, but it does inhibit the human and animal sorrow and suffering.

The link between the spiritual and the lower planes of the being is that which is called in the old Vedantic phraseology the *vijñāna* and which we may describe in our modern turn of language as the Truth-plane or the ideal mind or supermind. There the One and the Many meet and our being is freely open to the revealing light of the divine Truth and the inspiration of the divine Will and Knowledge. If we can break down the veil of the intellectual, emotional, sensational mind which our ordinary existence has built between us and the Divine, we can then take up through the Truth-mind all our mental, vital and physical experience and offer it up to the spiritual—this was the secret or mystic sense of the old Vedic "sacrifice"—to be converted into the terms of the infinite truth of Sachchidananda, and we can receive the powers and illuminations of the infinite Existence in forms of a divine knowledge, will and delight to be imposed on our mentality, vitality, physical existence till the lower members are transformed into the perfect vessel of the higher nature. This was the double Vedic movement of the descent and birth of the gods in the human creature and the ascent of the human powers that struggle towards the divine knowledge, power and delight and climb into the godheads, the result of which was the possession of the One, the infinite, the beatific existence, the union with God, the Immortality. By possession of this ideal plane we break down entirely the opposition of the lower and the higher existence, the false gulf created by the Ignorance between the finite and the Infinite, God and Nature, the One and the Many, open the gates of the Divine, fulfil the individual in the complete harmony of the cosmic consciousness and realise in the cosmic being the epiphany of the transcendent Sachchidananda. And these results, which obtained on the supramental plane itself or beyond, would be the highest perfection of the human being, we can attain to partially, in a very modified way, in a sort of mental figure by awakening into activity on the corresponding plane of the mental nature. We can get a luminous shadow of that perfect harmony and light. But this belongs to another part of our subject; it is the knowledge on which we must found our Yoga of self-perfection.

---

1. The Gita speaks of the Jiva as a portion of the Lord.
2. *Vijānataḥ*. Vijnana is the knowledge of the One and the Many, by which the Many are seen in the terms of the One, in the infinite unifying Truth, Right, Vast of the divine existence.
3. *jagatyāṁ jagat.* Isha Upanishad.

# ONENESS

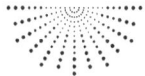

WHEN, then, by the withdrawal of the centre of consciousness from identification with the mind, life and body, one has discovered one's true self, discovered the oneness of that self with the pure, silent, immutable Brahman, discovered in the immutable, in the Akshara Brahman, that by which the individual being escapes from his own personality into the impersonal, the first movement of the Path of Knowledge has been completed. It is the sole that is absolutely necessary for the traditional aim of the Yoga of Knowledge, for immergence, for escape from cosmic existence, for release into the absolute and ineffable Parabrahman who is beyond all cosmic being. The seeker of this ultimate release may take other realisations on his way, may realise the Lord of the universe, the Purusha who manifests Himself in all creatures, may arrive at the cosmic consciousness, may know and feel his unity with all beings; but these are only stages or circumstances of his journey, results of the unfolding of his soul as it approaches nearer the ineffable goal. To pass beyond them all is his supreme object. When on the other hand, having attained to the freedom and the silence and the peace, we resume possession by the cosmic consciousness of the active as well as the silent Brahman and can securely live in the divine freedom as well as rest in it, we have completed the second movement of the Path by which the integrality of self-knowledge becomes the station of the liberated soul.

The soul thus possesses itself in the unity of Sachchidananda upon all the manifest planes of its own being. This is the characteristic of the integral knowledge that it unifies all in Sachchidananda because not only is Being one in itself, but it is one everywhere, in all its poises and in every aspect, in its utmost appearance of multiplicity as in its utmost appearance of oneness. The traditional knowledge while it admits this truth in theory, yet reasons practically as if the oneness were not equal everywhere or could not be equally realised in all. It finds it in the unmanifest Absolute, but not so much in the manifestation, finds it purer in the Impersonal than in the Personal, complete in the Nirguna, not so complete in the Saguna, satisfyingly present in the silent and inactive Brahman, not so satisfyingly present in the active. Therefore it places all these other terms of the Absolute below their opposites in the scale of ascent and urges their final rejection as if it were indispensable to the utter realisation. The integral knowledge makes no such division; it arrives at a different kind of absoluteness in its vision of the unity. It finds the same oneness in the Unmanifest and the Manifest, in the Impersonal and the Personal, in Nirguna and Saguna, in the infinite depths of the universal silence and the infinite largeness of the universal action. It finds the same absolute oneness in the Purusha and the Prakriti; in the divine Presence and the works of the divine Power and Knowledge; in the eternal manifestness of the one Purusha and the constant manifestation of the many Purushas; in the inalienable unity of Sachchidananda keeping constantly real to itself its own manifold oneness and in the apparent divisions of mind, life and body in which oneness is constantly, if secretly real and constantly seeks to be realised. All unity is to it an intense, pure and infinite realisation, all difference an abundant, rich and boundless realisation of the same divine and eternal Being.

The complete realisation of unity is therefore the essence of the integral knowledge and of the integral Yoga. To know Sachchidananda one in Himself and one in all His manifestation is the basis of knowledge; to make that vision of oneness real to the consciousness in its status and in its action and to become that by merging the sense of separate individuality in the sense of unity with the Being and with all beings is its effectuation in Yoga of knowledge; to live, think, feel, will and act in that sense of unity is its effectuation in the individual being and the individual life. This realisation of oneness and this practice of oneness in difference is the whole of the Yoga.

Sachchidananda is one in Himself in whatever status or whatever plane of existence. We have therefore to make that the basis of all effectuation whether of consciousness or force or being, whether of knowledge or will or delight. We have, as we have seen, to live in the consciousness of the Absolute transcendent and of the Absolute manifested in all relations, impersonal and manifest as all personalities, beyond all qualities and rich in infinite quality, a silence out of which the eternal Word creates, a divine calm and peace possessing itself in infinite joy and activity. We have to find Him knowing all, sanctioning all, governing all, containing, upholding and informing all as the Purusha and at the same time executing all knowledge, will and formation as Prakriti. We have to see Him as one Existence, Being gathered in itself and Being displayed in all existences; as one Consciousness concentrated in the unity of its existence, extended in universal nature and many-centred in innumerable beings; one Force static in its repose of self-gathered consciousness and dynamic in its activity of extended consciousness; one Delight blissfully aware of its featureless infinity and blissfully aware of all feature and force and forms as itself; one creative knowledge and governing Will, supramental, originative and determinative of all minds, lives and bodies; one Mind containing all mental beings and constituting all their mental activities; one Life active in all living beings and generative of their vital activities; one substance constituting all forms and objects as the visible and sensible mould in which mind and life manifest and act just as one pure existence is that ether in which all Conscious-Force and Delight exist unified and find themselves variously. For these are the seven principles of the manifest being of Sachchidananda.

The integral Yoga of knowledge has to recognise the double nature of this manifestation,—for there is the higher nature of Sachchidananda in which He is found and the lower nature of mind, life and body in which He is veiled,—and to reconcile and unite the two in the oneness of the illumined realisation. We have not to leave them separate so that we live a sort of double life, spiritual within or above, mental and material in our active and earthly living; we have to re-view and remould the lower living in the light, force and joy of the higher reality. We have to realise Matter as a sense-created mould of Spirit, a vehicle for all manifestation of the light, force and joy of Sachchidananda in the highest conditions of terrestrial being and activity. We have to see Life as a channel for the infinite Force divine and break the barrier of a sense-created and mind-created farness and division from it so that that divine Power may take possession of and direct and change all our life-activities until our vitality transfigured ceases in the end to be the limited life-force which now supports mind and body and becomes a figure of the all-blissful conscious-force of Sachchidananda. We have similarly to change our sensational and emotional mentality into a play of the divine Love and universal Delight; and we have to surcharge the intellect which seeks to know and will in us with the light of the divine Knowledge-Will until it is transformed into a figure of that higher and sublime activity.

This transformation cannot be complete or really executed without the awakening of the truth-mind which corresponds in the mental being to the Supermind and is capable of receiving mentally its illuminations. By the opposition of Spirit and Mind without the free opening of this intermediate power the two natures, higher and lower, stand divided, and though there may be communication and influence or the catching up of the lower into the higher in a sort of luminous or ecstatic trance, there cannot be a full and perfect transfiguration of the lower nature. We may feel imperfectly by the emotional mind, we may have a sense by the sense-mind or a conception and perception by the intelligent mind of the Spirit present in Matter and all its forms, the divine Delight present in all emotion and sensation, the divine Force behind all life-activities; but the lower will still keep its own nature and limit and divide in its action and modify in its character the influence from above. Even when that influence assumes its highest, widest, intensest power, it will be irregular and disorderly in activity and perfectly realised only in calm and stillness; we shall be subject to reactions and periods of obscuration when it is withdrawn from us; we shall be apt to forget it in the stress of ordinary life and its outward touches and the siege of its dualities and to be fully possessed of it only when alone with ourselves and God or else only in moments or periods of a heightened exaltation and ecstasy. For our mentality, a restricted instrument moving in a limited field and seizing things by fragments and parcels, is necessarily shifting, restless and mutable; it can find steadiness only by limiting its field of action and fixity only by cessation and repose.

Our direct truth-perceptions on the other hand come from that Supermind,—a Will that knows and a Knowledge that effects,—which creates universal order out of infinity. Its awakening into action brings down, says the Veda, the unrestricted downpour of the rain of heaven,— the full flowing of the seven rivers from a superior sea of light and power and joy. It reveals Sachchidananda. It reveals the Truth behind the scattered and ill-combined suggestions of our mentality and makes each to fall into its place in the unity of the Truth behind; thus it can transform the half-light of our minds into a certain totality of light. It reveals the Will behind all the devious and imperfectly regulated strivings of our mental will and emotional wishes and vital effort and makes each to fall into its place in the unity of the luminous Will behind; thus it can transform the half-obscure struggle of our life and mind into a certain totality of ordered force. It reveals the delight for which each of our sensations and emotions is groping and from which they fall back in movements of partially grasped satisfaction or of dissatisfaction, pain, grief or indifference, and makes each take its place in the unity of the universal delight behind; thus it can transform the conflict of our dualised emotions and sensations into a certain totality of serene, yet profound and powerful love and delight. Moreover, revealing the universal action, it shows the truth of being out of which each of its movements arises and to which each progresses, the force of effectuation which each carries with it and the delight of being for which and from which each is born, and it relates all to the universal being, consciousness, force and delight of Sachchidananda. Thus it harmonises for us all the oppositions, divisions, contrarieties of existence and shows us in them the One and the Infinite. Uplifted into this supramental light, pain and pleasure and indifference begin to be converted into joy of the one self-existent Delight; strength and weakness, success and failure turn into powers of the one self-effective Force and Will; truth and error, knowledge and ignorance change into light of the one infinite self-awareness and universal knowledge; increase of being and diminution of being, limitation and the overcoming of limitation are transfigured into waves of the one self-realising conscious existence. All our life as well as all our essential being is transformed into the possession of Sachchidananda.

By way of this integral knowledge we arrive at the unity of the aims set before themselves by the three paths of knowledge, works and devotion. Knowledge aims at the realisation of true self-existence; works are directed to the realisation of the divine Conscious-Will which secretly governs all works; devotion yearns for the realisation of the Bliss which enjoys as the Lover all beings and all existences,—Sat, Chit-Tapas and Ananda. Each therefore aims at possessing Sachchidananda through one or other aspect of his triune divine nature. By Knowledge we arrive always at our true, eternal, immutable being, the self-existent which every "I" in the universe obscurely represents, and we abrogate difference in the great realisation, So Aham, I am He, while we arrive also at our identity with all other beings.

But at the same time the integral knowledge gives us the awareness of that infinite existence as the conscious-force which creates and governs the worlds and manifests itself in their works; it reveals the Self-existent in his universal conscious-will as the Lord, the Ishwara. It enables us to unite our will with His, to realise His will in the energies of all existences and to perceive the fulfilment of these energies of others as part of our own universal self-fulfilment. Thus it removes the reality of strife and division and opposition and leaves only their appearances. By that knowledge therefore we arrive at the possibility of a divine action, a working which is personal to our nature, but impersonal to our being, since it proceeds from That which is beyond our ego and acts only by its universal sanction. We proceed in our works with equality, without bondage to works and their results, in unison with the Highest, in unison with the universal, free from separate responsibility for our acts and therefore unaffected by their reactions. This which we have seen to be the fulfilment of the path of Works becomes thus an annexe and result of the path of Knowledge.

The integral knowledge again reveals to us the Self-existent as the All-blissful who, as Sachchidananda manifesting the world, manifesting all beings, accepts their adoration, even as He accepts their works of aspiration and their seekings of knowledge, leans down to them and drawing them to Himself takes all into the joy of His divine being. Knowing Him as our divine Self, we become one with Him, as the lover and beloved become one, in the ecstasy of that embrace. Knowing Him too in all beings, perceiving the glory and beauty and joy of the Beloved everywhere, we transform our souls into a passion of universal delight and a wideness and joy of universal love. All this which, as we shall find, is the summit of the path of Devotion, becomes also an annexe and result of the path of Knowledge.

Thus by the integral knowledge we unify all things in the One. We take up all the chords of the universal music, strains sweet or discordant, luminous in their suggestion or obscure, powerful or faint, heard or suppressed, and find them all changed and reconciled in the indivisible harmony of Sachchidananda. The Knowledge brings also the Power and the Joy. "How shall he be deluded, whence shall he have sorrow who sees everywhere the Oneness?"

# THE SOUL AND NATURE

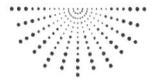

THIS IS the result of the integral knowledge taken in its mass; its work is to gather up the different strands of our being into the universal oneness. If we are to possess perfectly the world in our new divinised consciousness as the Divine himself possesses it, we have to know also each thing in its absoluteness, first by itself, secondly in its union with all that completes it; for so has the Divine imaged out and seen its being in the world. To see things as parts, as incomplete elements is a lower analytic knowledge. The Absolute is everywhere; it has to be seen and found everywhere. Every finite is an infinite and has to be known and sensed in its intrinsic infiniteness as well as in its surface finite appearance. But so to know the world, so to perceive and experience it, it is not enough to have an intellectual idea or imagination that so it is; a certain divine vision, divine sense, divine ecstasy is needed, an experience of union of ourselves with the objects of our consciousness. In that experience not only the Beyond but all here, not only the totality, the All in its mass, but each thing in the All becomes to us our self, God, the Absolute and Infinite, Sachchidananda. This is the secret of complete delight in God's world, complete satisfaction of the mind and heart and will, complete liberation of the consciousness. It is the supreme experience at which art and poetry and all the various efforts of subjective and objective knowledge and all desire and effort to possess and enjoy objects are trying more or less obscurely to arrive;

their attempt to seize the forms and properties and qualities of things is only a first movement which cannot give the deepest satisfaction unless by seizing them perfectly and absolutely they get the sense of the infinite reality of which these are the outer symbols. To the rational mind and the ordinary sense-experience this may well seem only a poetic fancy or a mystic hallucination; but the absolute satisfaction and sense of illumination which it gives and alone can give is really a proof of its greater validity; we get by that a ray from the higher consciousness and the diviner sense into which our subjective being is intended eventually, if we will only allow it, to be transfigured.

We have seen that this applies to the highest principles of the Divine Being. Ordinarily, the discriminating mind tells us that only what is beyond all manifestation is absolute, only the formless Spirit is infinite, only the timeless, spaceless, immutable, immobile Self in its repose is absolutely real; and if we follow and are governed in our endeavour by this conception, that is the subjective experience at which we shall arrive, all else seeming to us false or only relatively true. But if we start from the larger conception, a completer truth and a wider experience open to us. We perceive that the immutability of the timeless, spaceless existence is an absolute and an infinite, but that also the conscious-force and the active delight of the divine Being in its all-blissful possession of the outpouring of its powers, qualities, self-creations is an absolute and an infinite,—and indeed the same absolute and infinite, so much the same that we can enjoy simultaneously, equally the divine timeless calm and peace and the divine time-possessing joy of activity, freely, infinitely, without bondage or the lapse into unrest and suffering. So too we can have the same experience of all the principles of this activity which in the Immutable are self-contained and in a sense drawn in and concealed, in the cosmic are expressed and realise their infinite quality and capacity.

The first of these principles in importance is the duality—which resolves itself into a unity—of Purusha and Prakriti of which we have had occasion to speak in the Yoga of Works, but which is of equal importance for the Yoga of Knowledge. This division was made most clearly by the old Indian philosophies; but it bases itself upon the eternal fact of practical duality in unity upon which the world-manifestation is founded. It is given different names according to our view of the universe. The Vedantins spoke of the Self and Maya, meaning according to their predilections by the Self the Immutable and by Maya the power the Self has of imposing on itself the cosmic illusion, or by the Self the

Divine Being and by Maya the nature of conscious-being and the conscious-force by which the Divine embodies himself in soul-forms and forms of things. Others spoke of Ishwara and Shakti, the Lord and His force, His cosmic power. The analytic philosophy of the Sankhyas affirmed their eternal duality without any possibility of oneness, accepting only relations of union and separation by which the cosmic action of Prakriti begins, proceeds or ceases for the Purusha; for the Purusha is an inactive conscious existence,—it is the Soul the same in itself and immutable forever,—Prakriti the active force of Nature which by its motion creates and maintains and by its sinking into rest dissolves the phenomenon of the cosmos. Leaving aside these philosophical distinctions, we come to the original psychological experience from which all really take their start, that there are two elements in the existence of living beings, of human beings at least if not of all cosmos,—a dual being, Nature and the soul.

This duality is self-evident. Without any philosophy at all, by the mere force of experience it is what we can all perceive, although we may not take the trouble to define. Even the most thoroughgoing materialism which denies the soul or resolves it into a more or less illusory result of natural phenomena acting upon some ill-explained phenomenon of the physical brain which we call consciousness or the mind, but which is really no more than a sort of complexity of nervous spasms, cannot get rid of the practical fact of this duality. It does not matter at all how it came about; the fact is not only there, it determines our whole existence, it is the one fact which is really important to us as human beings with a will and an intelligence and a subjective existence which makes all our happiness and our suffering. The whole problem of life resolves itself into this one question,—"What are we to do with this soul and nature set face to face with each other,—we who have as one side of our existence this Nature, this personal and cosmic activity, which tries to impress itself upon the soul, to possess, control, determine it, and as the other side this soul which feels that in some mysterious way it has a freedom, a control over itself, a responsibility for what it is and does, and tries therefore to turn upon Nature, its own and the world's, and to control, possess, enjoy, or even, it may be, reject and escape from her?" In order to answer that question we have to know,—to know what the soul can do, to know what it can do with itself, to know too what it can do with Nature and the world. The whole of human philosophy, religion, science is really nothing but an attempt to get at the right data upon which it will be possible to answer the question and solve, as satisfactorily as our knowledge will allow, the problem of our existence.

The hope of a complete escape from our present strife with and subjection to our lower and troubled nature and existence arises when we perceive what religion and philosophy affirm, but modern thought has tried to deny, that there are two poises of our soul-existence, a lower, troubled and subjected, a higher, supreme, untroubled and sovereign, one vibrant in Mind, the other tranquil in Spirit. The hope not only of an escape, but of a completely satisfying and victorious solution comes when we perceive what some religions and philosophies affirm, but others seem to deny, that there is also in the dual unity of soul and nature a lower, an ordinary human status and a higher, a divine; for it is in the divine alone that the conditions of the duality stand reversed; there the soul becomes that which now it only struggles and aspires to be, master of its nature, free and by union with the Divine possessor also of the world-nature. According to our idea of these possibilities will be the solution we shall attempt to realise.

Involved in mind, possessed by the ordinary phenomenon of mental thought, sensation, emotion, reception of the vital and physical impacts of the world and mechanical reaction to them, the soul is subject to Nature. Even its will and intelligence are determined by its mental nature, determined even more largely by the mental nature of its environment which acts upon, subtly as well as overtly, and overcomes the individual mentality. Thus its attempt to regulate, to control, to determine its own experience and action is pursued by an element of illusion, since when it thinks it is acting, it is really Nature that is acting and determining all it thinks, wills and does. If there were not this constant knowledge in it that it is, that it exists in itself, is not the body or life but something other which at least receives and accepts the cosmic experience if it does not determine it, it would be compelled in the end to suppose that Nature is all and the soul an illusion. This is the conclusion modern Materialism affirms and to that nihilistic Buddhism arrived; the Sankhyas, perceiving the dilemma, solved it by saying that the soul in fact only mirrors Nature's determinations and itself determines nothing, is not the lord, but can by refusing to mirror them fall back into eternal immobility and peace. There are too the other solutions which arrive at the same practical conclusion, but from the other end, the spiritual; for they affirm either that Nature is an illusion or that both the soul and Nature are impermanent and they point us to a state beyond in which their duality has no existence; either they cease by the extinction of both in something permanent and ineffable or their discordances end by the exclusion of the active principle altogether. Though they do not satisfy humanity's larger hope and deep-seated impulse and aspiration, these are valid solutions so far as they go; for they arrive at an Absolute in itself or at the separate absolute of the soul, even if they reject the many rapturous infinities of the Absolute which the true possession of Nature by the soul in its divine existence offers to the eternal seeker in man.

Uplifted into the Spirit the soul is no longer subject to Nature; it is above this mental activity. It may be above it in detachment and aloofness, *udāsīna*, seated above and indifferent, or attracted by and lost in the absorbing peace or bliss of its undifferentiated, its concentrated spiritual experience of itself; we must then transcend by a complete renunciation of Nature and cosmic existence, not conquer by a divine and sovereign possession. But the Spirit, the Divine is not only above Nature; it is master of Nature and cosmos; the soul rising into its spiritual poise must at least be capable of the same mastery by its unity with the Divine. It must be capable of controlling its own nature not only in calm or by forcing it to repose, but with a sovereign control of its play and activity.

To arrive by an intense spirituality at the absolute of the soul is our possibility on one side of our dual existence; to enjoy the absolute of Nature and of everything in Nature is our possibility on the other side of this eternal duality. To unify these highest aspirations in a divine possession of God and ourselves and the world, should be our happy completeness. In the lower poise this is not possible because the soul acts through the mind and the mind can only act individually and fragmentarily in a contented obedience or a struggling subjection to that universal Nature through which the divine knowledge and the divine Will are worked out in the cosmos. But the Spirit is in possession of knowledge and will, of which it is the source and cause and not a subject; therefore in proportion as the soul assumes its divine or spiritual being, it assumes also control of the movements of its nature. It becomes, in the ancient language, Swarat, free and a self-ruler over the kingdom of its own life and being. But also it increases in control over its environment, its world.

This it can only do entirely by universalising itself; for it is the divine and universal will that it must express in its action upon the world. It must first extend its consciousness and see the universe in itself instead of being like the mind limited by the physical, vital, sensational, emotional, intellectual outlook of the little divided personality. It must accept the world-truths, the world-energies, the world-tendencies, the world-purposes as its own instead of clinging to its own intellectual ideas, desires and endeavours, preferences, objects, intentions, impulses; these, so far as they remain, must be harmonised with the universal. It must then submit its knowledge and will at their very source to the divine Knowledge and the divine Will and so arrive through submission at immergence, losing its personal light in the divine Light and its personal initiative in the divine initiative. To be first in tune with the Infinite, in harmony with the Divine, and then to be unified with the Infinite, taken into the Divine is its condition of perfect strength and mastery, and this is precisely the very nature of the spiritual life and the spiritual existence.

The distinction made in the Gita between the Purusha and the Prakriti gives us the clue to the various attitudes which the soul can adopt towards Nature in its movement towards perfect freedom and rule. The Purusha is, says the Gita, witness, upholder, source of the sanction, knower, lord, enjoyer; Prakriti executes, it is the active principle and must have an operation corresponding to the attitude of the Purusha. The soul may assume, if it wishes, the poise of the pure witness, *sākṣī*; it may look on at the action of Nature as a thing from which it stands apart; it watches, but does not itself participate. We have seen the importance of this quietistic capacity; it is the basis of the movement of withdrawal by which we can say of everything,—body, life, mental action, thought, sensation, emotion,—"This is Prakriti working in the life, mind and body, it is not myself, it is not even mine," and thus come to the soul's separation from these things and to their quiescence. This may, therefore, be an attitude of renunciation or at least of non-participation, tamasic, with a resigned and inert endurance of the natural action so long as it lasts, rajasic, with a disgust, aversion and recoil from it, sattwic, with a luminous intelligence of the soul's separateness and the peace and joy of aloofness and repose; but also it may be attended by an equal and impersonal delight as of a spectator at a show, joyous but unattached and ready to rise up at any moment and as joyfully depart. The attitude of the Witness at its highest is the absolute of unattachment and freedom from affection by the phenomena of the cosmic existence.

As the pure Witness, the soul refuses the function of up-holder or sustainer of Nature. The upholder, *bhartā*, is another, God or Force or Maya, but not the soul, which only admits the reflection of the natural action upon its watching consciousness, but not any responsibility for maintaining or continuing it. It does not say "All this is in me and maintained by me, an activity of my being," but at the most "This is imposed on me, but really external to myself." Unless there is a clear and real duality in existence, this cannot be the whole truth of the matter; the soul is the upholder also, it supports in its being the energy which unrolls the spectacle of the cosmos and which conducts its energies. When the Purusha accepts this upholding, it may do it still passively and without attachment, feeling that it contributes the energy, but not that it controls and determines it. The control is another, God or Force or the very nature of Maya; the soul only upholds indifferently so long as it must, so long perhaps as the force of its past sanction and interest in the energy continues and refuses to be exhausted. But if the attitude of the upholder is fully accepted, an important step forward has been taken towards identification with the active Brahman and his joy of cosmic being. For the Purusha has become the active giver of the sanction.

In the attitude of the Witness there is also a kind of sanction, but it is passive, inert and has no kind of absoluteness about it; but if he consents entirely to uphold, the sanction has become active, even though the soul may do no more than consent to reflect, support and thereby maintain in action all the energies of Prakriti. It may refuse to determine, to select, believing that it is God or Force itself or some Knowledge-Will that selects and determines, and the soul only a witness and upholder and thereby giver of the sanction, *anumantā*, but not the possessor and the director of the knowledge and the will, *jñātā īśvaraḥ*. Then there is a general sanction in the form of an active up-holding of whatever is determined by God or universal Will, but there is not an active determination. But if the soul habitually selects and rejects in what is offered to it, it determines; the relatively passive has become an entirely active sanction and is on the way to be an active control.

This it becomes when the soul accepts its complete function as the knower, lord and enjoyer of Nature. As the knower the soul possesses the knowledge of the force that acts and determines, it sees the values of being which are realising themselves in cosmos, it is in the secret of Fate. For the force that acts is itself determined by the knowledge which is its origin and the source and standardiser of its valuations and effectuations of values. Therefore in proportion as the soul becomes again the knower, it gets the capacity of becoming also the controller of the action whether by spiritual force alone or by that force figuring itself in mental and physical activities. There may be in our soul life a perfect spiritual knowledge and understanding not only of all our internal activities but of all the unrolling of things, events, human, animal, natural activities around us, the world-vision of the Rishi. This may not be attended by an active putting forth of power upon the world, though that is seldom entirely absent; for the Rishi is not uninterested in the world or in his fellow-creatures, but one with them by sympathy or by accepting all creatures as his own self in many minds and bodies. The old forest-dwelling anchorites even are described continually as busily engaged in doing good to all creatures. This can only be done in the spiritual realisation, not by an effort, for effort is a diminution of freedom, but by a spiritual influence or by a spiritual mastery over the minds of men and the workings of Nature, which reflects the divine effective immanence and the divine effective mastery.

Nor can it do this without becoming the active enjoyer, *bhoktā*. In the lower being the enjoyment is of a twofold kind, positive and negative, which in the electricity of sensation translates itself into joy and suffering; but in the higher it is an actively equal enjoyment of the divine delight in self-manifestation. That enjoyment again may be limited to a silent spiritual delight or an integral divine joy possessing all things around us and all activities of all parts of our being.

There is no loss of freedom, no descent into an ignorant attachment. The man free in his soul is aware that the Divine is the lord of the action of Nature, that Maya is His Knowledge-Will determining and effecting all, that Force is the Will side of this double divine Power in which knowledge is always present and effectual. He is aware of himself also, even individually, as a centre of the divine existence,—a portion of the Lord, the Gita expresses it,—controlling so far the action of Nature which he views, upholds, sanctions, enjoys, knows and by the determinative power of knowledge controls. And when he universalises himself, his knowledge still reflects only the divine knowledge, his will effectuates only the divine will, he enjoys only the divine delight and not an ignorant personal satisfaction. Thus the Purusha preserves its freedom in its possession, renunciation of limited personality even in its representative enjoyment and delight of cosmic being. It has taken up fully in the higher poise the true relations of the soul and Nature.

Purusha and Prakriti in their union and duality arise from the being of Sachchidananda. Self-conscious existence is the essential nature of the Being; that is Sat or Purusha. The Power of self-aware existence, whether drawn into itself or acting in the works of its consciousness and force, its knowledge and its will, Chit and Tapas, Chit and its Shakti,—that is Prakriti. Delight of being, Ananda, is the eternal truth of the union of this conscious being and its conscious force whether absorbed in itself or else deployed in the inseparable duality of its two aspects. It unrolls the worlds as Prakriti and views them as Purusha; acts in them and upholds the action; executes works and gives the sanction without which the force of Nature cannot act; executes and controls the knowledge and the will and knows and controls the determinations of the knowledge-force and will-force; ministers to the enjoyment and enjoys;—all is the Soul possessor, observer, knower, lord of Nature and Nature expressing the being, executing the will, satisfying the self-knowledge, ministering to the delight of being of the soul. There we have, founded on the very nature of being, the supreme and the universal relation of Prakriti with Purusha. The relation in its imperfect, perverted or reverse terms is the world as we see it; but the perfect relation brings the absolute joy of the soul in itself and, based upon that, the absolute joy of the soul in Nature which is the divine fulfilment of world-existence.

# THE SOUL AND ITS LIBERATION

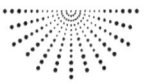

WE HAVE now to pause and consider to what this acceptance of the relations of Purusha and Prakriti commits us; for it means that the Yoga which we are pursuing has for end none of the ordinary aims of humanity. It neither accepts our earthly existence as it is, nor can be satisfied with some kind of moral perfection or religious ecstasy, with a heaven beyond or with some dissolution of our being by which we get satisfactorily done with the trouble of existence. Our aim becomes quite other; it is to live in the Divine, the Infinite, in God and not in any mere egoism and temporality, but at the same time not apart from Nature, from our fellow-beings, from earth and the mundane existence, any more than the Divine lives aloof from us and the world. He exists also in relation to the world and Nature and all these beings, but with an absolute and inalienable power, freedom and self-knowledge. Our liberation and perfection is to transcend ignorance, bondage and weakness and live in Him in relation to the world and Nature with the divine power, freedom and self-knowledge. For the highest relation of the Soul to existence is the Purusha's possession of Prakriti, when he is no longer ignorant and subject to his nature, but knows, transcends, enjoys and controls his manifested being and determines largely and freely what shall be his self-expression.

A oneness finding itself out in the variations of its own duality is the whole play of the soul with Nature in its cosmic birth and becoming.

One Sachchidananda everywhere, self-existent, illimitable, a unity indestructible by the utmost infinity of its own variations, is the original truth of being for which our knowledge seeks and to that our subjective existence eventually arrives. From that all other truths arise, upon that they are based, by that they are at every moment made possible and in that they in the end can know themselves and each other, are reconciled, harmonised and justified. All relations in the world, even to its greatest and most shocking apparent discords, are relations of something eternal to itself in its own universal existence; they are not anywhere or at any time collisions of disconnected beings who meet fortuitously or by some mechanical necessity of cosmic existence. Therefore to get back to this eternal fact of oneness is our essential act of self-knowledge; to live in it must be the effective principle of our inner possession of our being and of our right and ideal relations with the world. That is why we have had to insist first and foremost on oneness as the aim and in a way the whole aim of our Yoga of knowledge.

But this unity works itself out everywhere and on every plane by an executive or practical truth of duality. The Eternal is the one infinite conscious Existence, Purusha, and not something inconscient and mechanical; it exists eternally in its delight of the force of its own conscious being founded in an equilibrium of unity; but it exists also in the no less eternal delight of its force of conscious being at play with various creative self-experience in the universe. Just as we ourselves are or can become aware of being always something timeless, nameless, perpetual which we call our self and which constitutes the unity of all that we are, and yet simultaneously we have the various experience of what we do, think, will, create, become, such too is the self-awareness of this Purusha in the world. Only we, being at present limited and ego-bound mental individuals, have usually this experience in the ignorance and do not live in the self, but only look back at it or draw back to it from time to time, while the Eternal has it in His infinite self-knowledge, is eternally this self and looks from the fullness of self-being at all this self-experience. He does not like us, bound prisoners of the mind, conceive of His being as either a sort of indefinite result and sum or else a high contradiction of self-experience. The old philosophical quarrel between Being and Becoming is not possible to the eternal self-knowledge.

An active force of conscious-being which realises itself in its powers of self-experience, its powers of knowledge, will, self-delight, self-formulation with all their marvellous variations, inversions, conservations and conversions of energy, even perversions, is what we call Prakriti or Nature, in ourselves as in the cosmos. But behind this force of variation is the eternal equilibrium of the same force in an equal unity which supports impartially, governs even as it has originated the variations and directs them to whatever aim of its self-delight the Being, the Purusha, has conceived in its consciousness and determined by its will or power of consciousness. That is the divine Nature into unity with which we have to get back by our Yoga of self-knowledge. We have to become the Purusha, Sachchidananda, delighting in a divine individual possession of its Prakriti and no longer mental beings subject to our egoistic nature. For that is the real man, the supreme and integral self of the individual, and the ego is only a lower and partial manifestation of ourselves through which a certain limited and preparatory experience becomes possible and is for a time indulged. But this indulgence of the lower being is not our whole possibility; it is not the sole or crowning experience for which we exist as human beings even in this material world.

This individual being of ours is that by which ignorance is possible to self-conscious mind, but it is also that by which liberation into the spiritual being is possible and the enjoyment of divine immortality. It is not the Eternal in His transcendence or in His cosmic being who arrives at this immortality; it is the individual who rises into self-knowledge, in him it is possessed and by him it is made effective. All life, spiritual, mental or material, is the play of the soul with the possibilities of its nature; for without this play there can be no self-expression and no relative self-experience. Even, then, in our realisation of all as our larger self and in our oneness with God and other beings, this play can and must persist, unless we desire to cease from all self-expression and all but a tranced and absorbed self-experience. But then it is in the individual being that this trance or this liberated play is realised; the trance is this mental being's immersion in the sole experience of unity, the liberated play is the taking up of his mind into the spiritual being for the free realisation and delight of oneness. For the nature of the divine existence is to possess always its unity, but to possess it also in an infinite experience, from many standpoints, on many planes, through many conscious powers or selves of itself, individualities—in our limited intellectual language—of the one conscious being. Each one of us is one of these individualities. To stand away from God in limited ego, limited mind is to stand away from ourselves, to be unpossessed of our true individuality, to be the apparent and not the real individual; it is our power of ignorance. To be taken up into the divine Being and be aware of our spiritual, infinite and universal consciousness as that in which we now live, is to possess our supreme and integral self, our true individuality; it is our power of self-knowledge.

By knowing the eternal unity of these three powers of the eternal manifestation, God, Nature and the individual self, and their intimate necessity to each other, we come to understand existence itself and all that in the appearances of the world now puzzles our ignorance. Our self-knowledge abolishes none of these things, it abolishes only our ignorance and those circumstances proper to the ignorance which made us bound and subject to the egoistic determinations of our nature. When we get back to our true being, the ego falls away from us; its place is taken by our supreme and integral self, the true individuality. As this supreme self it makes itself one with all beings and sees all world and Nature in its own infinity. What we mean by this is simply that our sense of separate existence disappears into a consciousness of illimitable, undivided, infinite being in which we no longer feel bound to the name and form and the particular mental and physical determinations of our present birth and becoming and are no longer separate from anything or anyone in the universe. This was what the ancient thinkers called the Non-birth or the destruction of birth or Nirvana. At the same time we continue to live and act through our individual birth and becoming, but with a different knowledge and quite another kind of experience; the world also continues, but we see it in our own being and not as something external to it and other than ourselves. To be able to live permanently in this new consciousness of our real, our integral being is to attain liberation and enjoy immortality.

Here there comes in the complication of the idea that immortality is only possible after death in other worlds, upon higher planes of existence or that liberation must destroy all possibility of mental or bodily living and annihilate the individual existence for ever in an impersonal infinity. These ideas derive their strength from a certain justification in experience and a sort of necessity or upward attraction felt by the soul when it shakes off the compelling ties of mind and matter. It is felt that these ties are inseparable from all earthly living or from all mental existence. Death is the king of the material world, for life seems to exist here only by submission to death, by a constant dying; immortality has to be conquered here with difficulty and seems to be in its nature a rejection of all death and therefore of all birth into the material world. The field of immortality must be in some immaterial plane, in some heavens where either the body does not exist or else is different and only a form of the soul or a secondary circumstance. On the other hand, it is felt by those who would go beyond immortality even, that all planes and heavens are circumstances of the finite existence and the infinite self is void of all these things. They are dominated by a necessity to disappear into the impersonal and infinite and an inability to equate in any way the bliss of impersonal being with the soul's delight in its becoming. Philosophies have been invented which justify to the intellect this need of immersion and disappearance; but what is really important and decisive is the call of the Beyond, the need of the soul, its delight—in this case—in a sort of impersonal existence or non-existence. For what decides is the determining delight of the Purusha, the relation which it wills to establish with its Prakriti, the experience at which it arrives as the result of the line it has followed in the development of its individual self-experience among all the various possibilities of its nature. Our intellectual justifications are only the account of that experience which we give to the reason and the devices by which we help the mind to assent to the direction in which the soul is moving.

The cause of our world-existence is not, as our present experience induces us to believe, the ego; for the ego is only a result and a circumstance of our mode of world-existence. It is a relation which the many-souled Purusha has set up between individualised minds and bodies, a relation of self-defence and mutual exclusion and aggression in order to have among all the dependences of things in the world upon each other a possibility of independent mental and physical experience. But there can be no absolute independence upon these planes; impersonality which rejects all mental and physical becoming is therefore the only possible culmination of this exclusive movement: so only can an absolutely independent self-experience be achieved. The soul then seems to exist absolutely, independently in itself; it is free in the sense of the Indian word, *svādhīna*, dependent only on itself, not dependent upon God and other beings. Therefore in this experience God, personal self and other beings are all denied, cast away as distinctions of the ignorance. It is the ego recognising its own insufficiency and abolishing both itself and its contraries that its own essential instinct of independent self-experience may be accomplished; for it finds that its effort to achieve it by relations with God and others is afflicted throughout with a sentence of illusion, vanity and nullity. It ceases to admit them because by admitting them it becomes dependent on them; it ceases to admit its own persistence, because the persistence of ego means the admission of that which it tries to exclude as not-self, of the cosmos and other beings. The self-annihilation of the Buddhist is in its nature absolute exclusion of all that the mental being perceives; the self-immersion of the Adwaitin in his absolute being is the self-same aim differently conceived: both are a supreme self-assertion of the soul of its exclusive independence of Prakriti.

The experience which we first arrive at by the sort of short-cut to liberation which we have described as the movement of withdrawal, assists this tendency. For it is a breaking of the ego and a rejection of the habits of the mentality we now possess; for that is subject to matter and the physical senses and conceives of things only as forms, objects, external phenomena and as names which we attach to those forms. We are not aware directly of the subjective life of other beings except by analogy from our own and by inference or derivative perception based upon their external signs of speech, action, etc., which our minds translate into the terms of our own subjectivity. When we break out from ego and physical mind into the infinity of the spirit, we still see the world and others as the mind has accustomed us to see them, as names and forms; only in our new experience of the direct and superior reality of spirit, they lose that direct objective reality and that indirect subjective reality of their own which they had to the mind. They seem to be quite the opposite of the truer reality we now experience; our mentality, stilled and indifferent, no longer strives to know and make real to itself those intermediate terms which exist in them as in us and the knowledge of which has for its utility to bridge over the gulf between the spiritual self and the objective phenomena of the world. We are satisfied with the blissful infinite impersonality of a pure spiritual existence; nothing else and nobody else any longer matters to us. What the physical senses show to us and what the mind perceives and conceives about them and so imperfectly and transiently delights in, seems now unreal and worthless; we are not and do not care to be in possession of the intermediate truths of being through which these things are enjoyed by the One and possess for Him that value of His being and delight which makes, as we might say, cosmic existence a thing beautiful to Him and worth manifesting. We can no longer share in God's delight in the world; on the contrary it looks to us as if the Eternal had degraded itself by admitting into the purity of its being the gross nature of Matter or had falsified the truth of its being by imagining vain names and unreal forms. Or else if we perceive at all that delight, it is with a far-off detachment which prevents us from participating in it with any sense of intimate possession, or it is with an attraction to the superior delight of an absorbed and exclusive self-experience which does not allow us to stay any longer in these lower terms than we are compelled to stay by the continuance of our physical life and body.

But if either in the course of our Yoga or as the result of a free return of our realised Self upon the world and a free repossession of its Prakriti by the Purusha in us, we become conscious not only of the bodies and outward self-expression of others, but intimately of their inner being, their minds, their souls and that in them of which their own surface minds are not aware, then we see the real Being in them also and we see them as selves of our Self and not as mere names and forms. They become to us realities of the Eternal. Our minds are no longer subject to the delusion of trivial unworthiness or the illusion of unreality. The material life loses indeed for us its old absorbing value, but finds the greater value which it has for the divine Purusha; regarded no longer as the sole term of our becoming, but as merely having a subordinate value in relation to the higher terms of mind and spirit, it increases by that diminution instead of losing in value. We see that our material being, life, nature are only one poise of the Purusha in relation to its Prakriti and that their true purpose and importance can only be appreciated when they are seen not as a thing in itself, but as dependent on higher poises by which they are supported; from those superior relations they derive their meaning and, therefore, by conscious union with them they can fulfil all their valid tendencies and aims. Life then becomes justified to us and no longer stultified by the possession of liberated self-knowledge.

This larger integral knowledge and freedom liberates in the end and fulfils our whole existence. When we possess it, we see why our existence moves between these three terms of God, ourselves and the world; we no longer see them or any of them in opposition to each other, inconsistent, incompatible, nor do we on the other hand regard them as terms of our ignorance which all disappear at last into a pure impersonal unity. We perceive their necessity as terms rather of our self-fulfilment which preserve their value after liberation or rather find then only their real value. We have no longer the experience of our existence as exclusive of the other existences which make up by our relations with them our experience of the world; in this new consciousness they are all contained in ourselves and we in them. They and we are no longer so many mutually exclusive egos each seeking its own independent fulfilment or self-transcendence and ultimately aiming at nothing else; they are all the Eternal and the self in each secretly embraces all in itself and seeks in various ways to make that higher truth of its unity apparent and effective in its terrestrial being. Not mutual exclusiveness, but mutual inclusiveness is the divine truth of our individuality, love the higher law and not an independent self-fulfilment.

The Purusha who is our real being is always independent and master of Prakriti and at this independence we are rightly seeking to arrive; that is the utility of the egoistic movement and its self-transcendence, but its right fulfilment is not in making absolute the ego's principle of independent existence, but in arriving at this other highest poise of the Purusha with regard to its Prakriti. There there is transcendence of Nature, but also possession of Nature, perfect fulfilment of our individuality, but also perfect fulfilment of our relations with the world and with others. Therefore an individual salvation in heavens beyond careless of the earth is not our highest objective; the liberation and self-fulfilment of others is as much our own concern,—we might almost say, our divine self-interest,— as our own liberation. Otherwise our unity with others would have no effective meaning. To conquer the lures of egoistic existence in this world is our first victory over ourselves; to conquer the lure of individual happiness in heavens beyond is our second victory; to conquer the highest lure of escape from life and a self-absorbed bliss in the impersonal infinity is the last and greatest victory. Then are we rid of all individual exclusiveness and possessed of our entire spiritual freedom.

The state of the liberated soul is that of the Purusha who is for ever free. Its consciousness is a transcendence and an all-comprehending unity. Its self-knowledge does not get rid of all the terms of self-knowledge, but unifies and harmonises all things in God and in the divine nature. The intense religious ecstasy which knows only God and ourselves and shuts out all else, is only to it an intimate experience which prepares it for sharing in the embrace of the divine Love and Delight around all creatures. A heavenly bliss which unites God and ourselves and the blest, but enables us to look with a remote indifference on the unblest and their sufferings is not possible to the perfect soul; for these also are its selves; free individually from suffering and ignorance, it must naturally turn to draw them also towards its freedom. On the other hand any absorption in the relations between self and others and the world to the exclusion of God and the Beyond is still more impossible, and therefore it cannot be limited by the earth or even by the highest and most altruistic relations of man with man. Its activity or its culmination is not to efface and utterly deny itself for the sake of others, but to fulfil itself in God-possession, freedom and divine bliss that in and by its fulfilment others too may be fulfilled. For it is in God alone, by the possession of the Divine only that all the discords of life can be resolved, and therefore the raising of men towards the Divine is in the end the one effective way of helping mankind. All the other activities and realisations of our self-experience have their use and power, but in the end these crowded side-tracks or these lonely paths must circle round to converge into the wideness of the integral way by which the liberated soul transcends all, embraces all and becomes the promise and the power of the fulfilment of all in their manifested being of the Divine.

# THE PLANES OF OUR EXISTENCE

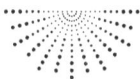

IF THE Purusha in us has thus to become by union with its highest self, the Divine Purusha, the knower, lord, free enjoyer of its Prakriti, it cannot be done, evidently, by dwelling on the present plane of our being; for that is the material plane in which the reign of Prakriti is complete; there the divine Purusha is entirely hidden in the blinding surge of her activities, in the gross pomp of her workings, and the individual soul emerging from her involution of spirit in matter, subject in all its activities to its entangling in the material and vital instruments is unable to experience the divine freedom. What it calls its freedom and mastery, is only the subtle subjection of mind to Prakriti which is lighter indeed, nearer to the possibility of liberty and rule than the gross subjection of vital and material things like the animal, plant and metal, but is still not real freedom and mastery. Therefore we have had to speak of different planes of our consciousness and of the spiritual planes of the mental being; for if these did not exist, the liberation of the embodied being would have been impossible here on earth. He would have had to wait and at most to prepare himself for seeking it in other worlds and in a different kind of physical or spiritual embodiment less obstinately sealed in its shell of material experience.

In the ordinary Yoga of knowledge it is only necessary to recognise two planes of our consciousness, the spiritual and the materialised mental; the pure reason standing between these two views them both, cuts through the illusions of the phenomenal world, exceeds the materialised mental plane, sees the reality of the spiritual; and then the will of the individual Purusha unifying itself with this poise of knowledge rejects the lower and draws back to the supreme plane, dwells there, loses mind and body, sheds life from it and merges itself in the supreme Purusha, is delivered from individual existence. It knows that this is not the whole truth of our existence, which is much more complex; it knows there are many planes, but it disregards them or pays little attention to them because they are not essential to this liberation. They indeed rather hamper it, because to live on them brings new attractive psychical experiences, psychical enjoyments, psychical powers, a new world of phenomenal knowledge the pursuit of which creates stumbling-blocks in the way of its one object, immergence in Brahman, and brings a succession of innumerable way-side snares on the road which leads to God. But since we accept world-existence, and for us all world-existence is Brahman and full of the presence of God, these things can have no terrors for us; whatever dangers of distraction there may be, we have to face and overcome them. If the world and our own existence are so complex, we must know and embrace their complexities in order that our self-knowledge and our knowledge of the dealings of Purusha with its Prakriti may be complete. If there are many planes, we have to possess them all for the Divine, even as we seek to possess spiritually and transform our ordinary poise of mind, life and body.

The ancient knowledge in all countries was full of the search after the hidden truths of our being and it created that large field of practice and inquiry which goes in Europe by the name of occultism,—we do not use any corresponding word in the East, because these things do not seem to us so remote, mysterious and abnormal as to the occidental mentality; they are nearer to us and the veil between our normal material life and this larger life is much thinner. In India,[1] Egypt, Chaldea, China, Greece, the Celtic countries they have formed part of various Yogic systems and disciplines which had once a great hold everywhere, but to the modern mind have seemed mere superstition and mysticism, although the facts and experiences on which they are founded are quite as real in their own field and as much governed by intelligible laws of their own as the facts and experiences of the material world. It is not our intention here to plunge into this vast and difficult field of psychical knowledge.[2] But it becomes necessary now to deal with certain broad facts and principles which form its framework, for without them our Yoga of knowledge cannot be complete. We find that in the various systems the facts dealt with are always the same, but there are considerable differences of theoretic and practical arrangement, as is natural and inevitable in dealing with a subject so large and difficult. Certain things are here omitted, there made all-important, here understressed, there over-emphasised; certain fields of experience which are in one system held to be merely subordinate provinces, are in others treated as separate kingdoms. But I shall follow here consistently the Vedic and Vedantic arrangement of which we find the great lines in the Upanishads, first because it seems to me at once the simplest and most philosophical and more especially because it was from the beginning envisaged from the point of view of the utility of these various planes to the supreme object of our liberation. It takes as its basis the three principles of our ordinary being, mind, life and matter, the triune spiritual principle of Sachchidananda and the link principle of *vijñāna*, supermind, the free or spiritual intelligence, and thus arranges all the large possible poises of our being in a tier of seven planes,—sometimes regarded as five only, because, only the lower five are wholly accessible to us,—through which the developing being can rise to its perfection.

But first we must understand what we mean by planes of consciousness, planes of existence. We mean a general settled poise or world of relations between Purusha and Prakriti, between the Soul and Nature. For anything that we can call world is and can be nothing else than the working out of a general relation which a universal existence has created or established between itself, or let us say its eternal fact or potentiality and the powers of its becoming. That existence in its relations with and its experience of the becoming is what we call soul or Purusha, individual soul in the individual, universal soul in the cosmos; the principle and the powers of the becoming are what we call Nature or Prakriti. But since Being, conscious force and delight of being are always the three constituent terms of existence, the nature of a world is really determined by the way in which Prakriti is set to deal with these three primary things and the forms which it is allowed to give to them. For existence itself is and must always be the stuff of its own becoming; it must be shaped into the substance with which Force has to deal. Force again must be the power which works out that substance and works with it to whatever ends; Force is that which we ordinarily call Nature. Again the end, the object with which the worlds are created must be worked out by the consciousness inherent in all existence and all force and all their workings, and the object must be the possession of itself and of its delight of existence in the world. To that all the circumstances and aims of any world-existence must reduce themselves; it is existence developing its terms of being, its power of being, its conscious delight of being; if these are involved, their evolution; if they are veiled, their self-revelation.

Here the soul lives in a material universe; of that alone it is immediately conscious; the realisation of its potentialities in that is the problem with which it is concerned. But matter means the involution of the conscious delight of existence in self-oblivious force and in a self-dividing, infinitesimally disaggregated form of substance. Therefore the whole principle and effort of a material world must be the evolution of what is involved and the development of what is undeveloped. Here everything is shut up from the first in the violently working inconscient sleep of material force; therefore the whole aim of any material becoming must be the waking of consciousness out of the inconscient; the whole consummation of a material becoming must be the removal of the veil of matter and the luminous revelation of the entirely self-conscient Being to its own imprisoned soul in the becoming. Since Man is such an imprisoned soul, this luminous liberation and coming to self-knowledge must be his highest object and the condition of his perfection.

But the limitations of a material universe seem to be hostile to the proper accomplishment of this object which is yet so inevitably the highest aim of a mental being born into a physical body. First existence has formed itself here, fundamentally, as Matter; it has been objectivised, made sensible and concrete to its own self-experiencing conscious-force in the form of self-dividing material substance, and by the aggregation of this matter there has been built up for man a physical body separate, divided from others and subject to the fixed habits of process or, as we call them, the laws of inconscient material Nature. His force of being too is nature or Force working in matter, which has waked slowly out of inconscience to life and is always limited by form, always dependent on the body, always separated by it from the rest of Life and from other living beings, always hampered in its development, persistence, self-perfectioning by the laws of the Inconscience and the limitations of bodily living. Equally, his consciousness is a mentality emerging in a body and in a sharply individualised life; it is therefore limited in its workings and capacities and dependent on bodily organs of no great competence and on a very restricted vital force; it is separated from the rest of cosmic mind and shut out from the thoughts of other mental beings whose inner workings are a sealed book to man's physical mind except in so far as he can read them by the analogy of his own mentality and by their insufficient bodily signs and self-expressions. His consciousness is always falling back towards the inconscience in which a large part of it is always involved, his life towards death, his physical being towards disaggregation. His delight of being depends on the relations of this imperfect consciousness with its environment based upon physical sensations and the sense-mind, in other words on a limited mind trying to lay hold on a world external and foreign to it by means of a limited body, limited vital force, limited organs. Therefore its power for possession is limited, its force for delight is limited, and every touch of the world which exceeds its force, which that force cannot bear, cannot seize on, cannot assimilate and possess must turn to something else than delight, to pain, discomfort or grief. Or else it must be met by non-reception, insensibility, or, if received, put away by indifference. Moreover such delight of being as it possesses, is not possessed naturally and eternally like the self-delight of Sachchidananda, but by experience and acquisition in Time, and can therefore only be maintained and prolonged by repetition of experience and is in its nature precarious and transient.

All this means that the natural relations of Purusha to Prakriti in the material universe are the complete absorption of conscious being in the force of its workings, therefore the complete self-oblivion and self-ignorance of the Purusha, the complete domination of Prakriti and subjection of the soul to Nature. The soul does not know itself, it only knows, if anything, the workings of Prakriti. The emergence of the individual self-conscious soul in Man does not of itself abrogate these primary relations of ignorance and subjection. For this soul is living on a material plane of existence, a poise of Prakriti in which matter is still the chief determinant of its relations to Nature, and its consciousness being limited by Matter cannot be an entirely self-possessing consciousness. Even the universal soul, if limited by the material formula, could not be in entire possession of itself; much less can the individual soul to which the rest of existence becomes by bodily, vital and mental limitation and separation something external to it on which it is yet dependent for its life and its delight and its knowledge. These limitations of his power, knowledge, life, delight of existence are the whole cause of man's dissatisfaction with himself and the universe. And if the material universe were all and the material plane the only plane of his being, then man the individual Purusha could never arrive at perfection and self-fulfilment or indeed to any other life than that of the animals. There must be either worlds in which he is liberated from these incomplete and unsatisfactory relations of Purusha with Prakriti, or planes of his own being by ascending to which he can transcend them, or at the very least planes, worlds and higher beings from which he can receive or be helped to knowledge, powers, joys, a growth of his being otherwise impossible. All these things, the ancient knowledge asserts, exist,—other worlds, higher planes, the possibility of communication, of ascension, of growth by contact with and influence from that which is above him in the present scale of his realised being.

As there is a poise of the relations of Purusha with Prakriti in which Matter is the first determinant, a world of material existence, so there is another just above it in which Matter is not supreme, but rather Life-force takes its place as the first determinant. In this world forms do not determine the conditions of the life, but it is life which determines the form, and therefore forms are there much more free, fluid, largely and to our conceptions strangely variable than in the material world. This life-force is not inconscient material force, not even, except in its lowest movements, an elemental subconscient energy, but a conscious force of being which makes for formation, but much more essentially for enjoyment, possession, satisfaction of its own dynamic impulse. Desire and the satisfaction of impulse are therefore the first law of this world of sheer vital existence, this poise of relations between the soul and its nature in which the life-power plays with so much greater a freedom and capacity than in our physical living; it may be called the desire-world, for that is its principal characteristic. Moreover, it is not fixed in one hardly variable formula as physical life seems to be, but is capable of many variations of its poise, admits many sub-planes ranging from those which touch material existence and, as it were, melt into that, to those which touch at the height of the life-power the planes of pure mental and psychic existence and melt into them. For in Nature in the infinite scale of being there are no wide gulfs, no abrupt chasms to be overleaped, but a melting of one thing into another, a subtle continuity; out of that her power of distinctive experience creates the orderings, the definite ranges, the distinct gradations by which the soul variously knows and possesses its possibilities of world-existence. Again, enjoyment of one kind or another being the whole object of desire, that must be the trend of the desire-world; but since wherever the soul is not free,—and it cannot be free when subject to desire,—there must be the negative as well as the positive of all its experience, this world contains not only the possibility of large or intense or continuous enjoyments almost inconceivable to the limited physical mind, but also the possibility of equally enormous sufferings. It is here therefore that there are situated the lowest heavens and all the hells with the tradition and imagination of which the human mind has lured and terrified itself since the earliest ages. All human imaginations indeed correspond to some reality or real possibility, though they may in themselves be a quite inaccurate representation or couched in too physical images and therefore inapt to express the truth of supraphysical realities.

Nature being a complex unity and not a collection of unrelated phenomena, there can be no unbridgeable gulf between the material existence and this vital or desire world. On the contrary, they may be said in a sense to exist in each other and are at least interdependent to a certain extent. In fact, the material world is really a sort of projection from the vital, a thing which it has thrown out and separated from itself in order to embody and fulfil some of its desires under conditions other than its own, which are yet the logical result of its own most material longings. Life on earth may be said to be the result of the pressure of this life-world on the material, inconscient existence of the physical universe. Our own manifest vital being is also only a surface result of a larger and profounder vital being which has its proper seat on the life-plane and through which we are connected with the life-world. Moreover, the life-world is constantly acting upon us and behind everything in material existence there stand appropriate powers of the life-world; even the most crude and elemental have behind them elemental life-powers, elemental beings by which or by whom they are supported. The influences of the life-world are always pouring out on the material existence and producing there their powers and results which return again upon the life-world to modify it. From that the life-part of us, the desire-part is being always touched and influenced; there too are beneficent and malefic powers of good desire and evil desire which concern themselves with us even when we are ignorant of and unconcerned with them. Nor are these powers merely tendencies, inconscient forces, nor, except on the verges of Matter, subconscient, but conscious powers, beings, living influences. As we awaken to the higher planes of our existence, we become aware of them as friends or enemies, powers which seek to possess or which we can master, overcome, pass beyond and leave behind. It is this possible relation of the human being with the powers of the life-world which occupied to so large an extent European occultism, especially in the Middle Ages, as well as certain forms of Eastern magic and spiritualism. The "superstitions" of the past—much superstition there was, that is to say, much ignorant and distorted belief, false explanations and obscure and clumsy dealing with the laws of the beyond,—had yet behind them truths which a future Science, delivered from its sole preoccupation with the material world, may rediscover. For the supra-material is as much a reality as the existence of mental beings in the material universe.

But why then are we not normally aware of so much that is behind us and always pressing upon us? For the same reason that we are not aware of the inner life of our neighbour, although it exists as much as our own and is constantly exercising an occult influence upon us,—for a great part of our thoughts and feelings come into us from outside, from our fellow-men, both from individuals and from the collective mind of humanity; and for the same reason that we are not aware of the greater part of our own being which is subconscient or subliminal to our waking mind and is a ways influencing and in an occult manner determining our surface existence. It is because we use, normally, only our corporeal senses and live almost wholly in the body and the physical vitality and the physical mind, and it is not directly through these that the life-world enters into relations with us. That is done through other sheaths of our being,—so they are termed in the Upanishads,—other bodies, as they are called in a later terminology, the mental sheath or subtle body in which our true mental being lives and the life sheath or vital body which is more closely connected with the physical or food-sheath and forms with it the gross body of our complex existence. These possess powers, senses, capacities which are always secretly acting in us, are connected with and impinge upon our physical organs and the plexuses of our physical life and mentality. By self-development we can become aware of them, possess our life in them, get through them into conscious relation with the life-world and other worlds and use them also for a more subtle experience and more intimate knowledge of the truths, facts and happenings of even the material world itself. We can by this self-development live more or less fully on planes of our existence other than the material which is now all in all to us.

What has been said of the life-world applies with the necessary differences to still higher planes of the cosmic existence. For beyond that is a mental plane, a world of mental existence in which neither life, nor matter, but mind is the first determinant. Mind there is not determined by material conditions or by the life-force, but itself determines and uses them for its own satisfaction. There mind, that is to say, the psychical and the intellectual being, is free in a certain sense, free at least to satisfy and fulfil itself in a way hardly conceivable to our body-bound and life-bound mentality; for the Purusha there is the pure mental being and his relations with Prakriti are determined by that purer mentality, Nature there is mental rather than vital and physical. Both the life-world and indirectly the material are a projection from that, the result of certain tendencies of the mental Being which have sought a field, conditions, an arrangement of harmonies proper to themselves; and the phenomena of mind in this world may be said to be a result of the pressure of that plane first on the life-world and then on life in the material existence. By its modification in the life-world it creates in us the desire-mind; in its own right it awakes in us the purer powers of our psychical and intellectual existence. But our surface mentality is only a secondary result of a larger subliminal mentality whose proper seat is the mental plane. This world of mental existence also is constantly acting upon us and our world, has its powers and its beings, is related to us through our mental body. There we find the psychical and mental heavens to which the Purusha can ascend when it drops this physical body and can there sojourn till the impulse to terrestrial existence again draws it downward. Here too are many planes, the lowest converging upon and melting into the worlds below, the highest at the heights of the mind-power into the worlds of a more spiritual existence.

These highest worlds are therefore supramental; they belong to the principle of supermind, the free, spiritual or divine intelligence[3] or gnosis and to the triple spiritual principle of Sachchidananda. From them the lower worlds derive by a sort of fall of the Purusha into certain specific or narrow conditions of the play of the soul with its nature. But these also are divided from us by no unbridgeable gulf; they affect us through what are called the knowledge-sheath and the bliss-sheath, through the causal or spiritual body, and less directly through the mental body, nor are their secret powers absent from the workings of the vital and material existence. Our conscious spiritual being and our intuitive mind awaken in us as a result of the pressure of these highest worlds on the mental being in life and body. But this causal body is, as we may say, little developed in the majority of men and to live in it or to ascend to the supramental planes, as distinguished from corresponding sub-planes in the mental being, or still more to dwell consciously upon them is the most difficult thing of all for the human being. It can be done in the trance of Samadhi, but otherwise only by a new evolution of the capacities of the individual Purusha of which few are even willing to conceive. Yet is that the condition of the perfect self-consciousness by which alone the Purusha can possess the full conscious control of Prakriti; for there not even the mind determines, but the Spirit freely uses the lower differentiating principles as minor terms of its existence governed by the higher and reaching by them their own perfect capacity. That alone would be the perfect evolution of the involved and development of the undeveloped for which the Purusha has sought in the material universe, as if in a wager with itself, the conditions of the greatest difficulty.

---

1. For example, the Tantric in India.
2. We hope to deal with it hereafter; but our first concern in the *Arya* must be with spiritual and philosophical truths; it is only when these have been grasped that the approach to the psychical becomes safe and clear.
3. Called the *vijñāna* or *buddhi*, a word which may lead to some misunderstanding as it is also applied to the mental intelligence which is only a lower derivation from the divine gnosis.

# THE LOWER TRIPLE PURUSHA

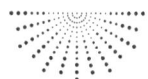

SUCH is the constituent principle of the various worlds of cosmic existence and the various planes of our being; they are as if a ladder plunging down into Matter and perhaps below it, rising up into the heights of the Spirit, even perhaps to the point at which existence escapes out of cosmic being into ranges of a supra-cosmic Absolute,—so at least it is averred in the world-system of the Buddhists. But to our ordinary materialised consciousness all this does not exist because it is hidden from us by our preoccupation with our existence in a little corner of the material universe and with the petty experiences of the little hour of time which is represented by our life in a single body upon this earth. To that consciousness the world is a mass of material things and forces thrown into some kind of shape and harmonised into a system of regulated movements by a number of fixed self-existent laws which we have to obey, by which we are governed and circumscribed and of which we have to get the best knowledge we can so as to make the most of this one brief existence which begins with birth, ends with death and has no second recurrence. Our own being is a sort of accident or at least a very small and minor circumstance in the universal life of Matter or the eternal continuity of the workings of material Force. Somehow or other a soul or mind has come to exist in a body and it stumbles about among things and forces which it does not very well understand, at first preoccupied with the difficulty of managing to live in a dangerous and largely hostile world and then with the effort to understand its laws and use them so as to make life as tolerable or as happy as possible so long as it lasts. If we were really nothing more than such a minor movement of individualised mind in Matter, existence would have nothing more to offer us; its best part would be at most this struggle of an ephemeral intellect and will with eternal Matter and with the difficulties of Life supplemented and eased by a play of imagination and by the consoling fictions presented to us by religion and art and all the wonders dreamed of by the brooding mind and restless fancy of man.

But because he is a soul and not merely a living body, man can never for long remain satisfied that this first view of his existence, the sole view justified by the external and objective facts of life, is the real truth or the whole knowledge: his subjective being is full of hints and inklings of realities beyond, it is open to the sense of infinity and immortality, it is easily convinced of other worlds, higher possibilities of being, larger fields of experience for the soul. Science gives us the objective truth of existence and the superficial knowledge of our physical and vital being; but we feel that there are truths beyond which possibly through the cultivation of our subjective being and the enlargement of its powers may come to lie more and more open to us. When the knowledge of this world is ours, we are irresistibly impelled to seek for the knowledge of other states of existence beyond, and that is the reason why an age of strong materialism and scepticism is always followed by an age of occultism, of mystical creeds, of new religions and profounder seekings after the Infinite and the Divine. The knowledge of our superficial mentality and the laws of our bodily life is not enough; it brings us always to all that mysterious and hidden depth of subjective existence below and behind of which our surface consciousness is only a fringe or an outer court. We come to see that what is present to our physical senses is only the material shell of cosmic existence and what is obvious in our superficial mentality is only the margin of immense continents which lie behind unexplored. To explore them must be the work of another knowledge than that of physical science or of a superficial psychology.

Religion is the first attempt of man to get beyond himself and beyond the obvious and material facts of his existence. Its first essential work is to confirm and make real to him his subjective sense of an Infinite on which his material and mental being depends and the aspiration of his soul to come into its presence and live in contact with it. Its function is to assure him too of that possibility of which he has always dreamed, but of which his ordinary life gives him no assurance, the possibility of transcending himself and growing out of bodily life and mortality into the joy of immortal life and spiritual existence. It also confirms in him the sense that there are worlds or planes of existence other than that in which his lot is now cast, worlds in which this mortality and this subjection to evil and suffering are not the natural state, but rather bliss of immortality is the eternal condition. Incidentally, it gives him a rule of mortal life by which he shall prepare himself for immortality. He is a soul and not a body and his earthly life is a means by which he determines the future conditions of his spiritual being. So much is common to all religions; beyond this we get from them no assured certainty. Their voices vary; some tell us that one life on earth is all we have in which to determine our future existence, deny the past immortality of the soul and assert only its future immortality, threaten it even with the incredible dogma of a future of eternal suffering for those who miss the right path, while others more large and rational affirm successive existences by which the soul grows into the knowledge of the Infinite with a complete assurance for all of ultimate arrival and perfection. Some present the Infinite to us as a Being other than ourselves with whom we can have personal relations, others as an impersonal existence into which our separate being has to merge; some therefore give us as our goal worlds beyond in which we dwell in the presence of the Divine, others a cessation of world-existence by immergence in the Infinite. Most invite us to bear or to abandon earthly life as a trial or a temporary affliction or a vanity and fix our hopes beyond; in some we find a vague hint of a future triumph of the Spirit, the Divine in the body, upon this earth, in the collective life of man, and so justify not only the separate hope and aspiration of the individual but the united and sympathetic hope and aspiration of the race. Religion in fact is not knowledge, but a faith and aspiration; it is justified indeed both by an imprecise intuitive knowledge of large spiritual truths and by the subjective experience of souls that have risen beyond the ordinary life, but in itself it only gives us the hope and faith by which we may be induced to aspire to the intimate possession of the hidden tracts and larger realities of the Spirit. That we turn always the few distinct truths and the symbols or the particular discipline of a religion into hard and fast dogmas, is a sign that as yet we are only infants in the spiritual knowledge and are yet far from the science of the Infinite.

Yet behind every great religion, behind, that is to say, its exoteric side of faith, hope, symbols, scattered truths and limiting dogmas, there is an esoteric side of inner spiritual training and illumination by which the hidden truths may be known, worked out, possessed. Behind every exoteric religion there is an esoteric Yoga, an intuitive knowledge to which its faith is the first step, inexpressible realities of which its symbols are the figured expression, a deeper sense for its scattered truths, mysteries of the higher planes of existence of which even its dogmas and superstitions are crude hints and indications. What Science does for our knowledge of the material world, replacing first appearances and uses by the hidden truths and as yet occult powers of its great natural forces and in our own minds beliefs and opinions by verified experience and a profounder understanding, Yoga does for the higher planes and worlds and possibilities of our being which are aimed at by the religions. Therefore all this mass of graded experience existing behind closed doors to which the consciousness of man may find, if it wills, the key, falls within the province of a comprehensive Yoga of knowledge, which need not be confined to the seeking after the Absolute alone or the knowledge of the Divine in itself or of the Divine only in its isolated relations with the individual human soul. It is true that the consciousness of the Absolute is the highest reach of the Yoga of knowledge and that the possession of the Divine is its first, greatest and most ardent object and that to neglect it for an inferior knowledge is to afflict our Yoga with inferiority or even frivolity and to miss or fall away from its characteristic object; but, the Divine in itself being known, the Yoga of knowledge may well embrace also the knowledge of the Divine in its relations with ourselves and the world on the different planes of our existence. To rise to the pure Self being steadfastly held to as the summit of our subjective self-uplifting, we may from that height possess our lower selves even to the physical and the workings of Nature which belong to them.

We may seek this knowledge on two sides separately, the side of Purusha, the side of Prakriti; and we may combine the two for the perfect possession of the various relations of Purusha and Prakriti in the light of the Divine. There is, says the Upanishad, a fivefold soul in man and the world, the microcosm and the macrocosm. The physical soul, self or being,—Purusha, Atman,—is that of which we are all at first conscious, a self which seems to have hardly any existence apart from the body and no action vital or even mental independent of it. This physical soul is present everywhere in material Nature; it pervades the body, actuates obscurely its movements and is the whole basis of its experiences; it informs all things even that are not mentally conscious. But in man this physical being has become vitalised and mentalised; it has received something of the law and capacities of the vital and mental being and nature. But its possession of them is derivative, superimposed, as it were, on its original nature and exercised under subjection to the law and action of the physical existence and its instruments. It is this dominance of our mental and vital parts by the body and the physical nature which seems at first sight to justify the theory of the materialists that mind and life are only circumstances and results of physical force and all their operations explicable by the activities of that force in the animal body. In fact entire subjection of the mind and the life to the body is the characteristic of an undeveloped humanity, as it is in an even greater degree of the infra-human animal. According to the theory of reincarnation those who do not get beyond this stage in the earthly life, cannot rise after death to the mental or higher vital worlds, but have to return from the confines of a series of physical planes to increase their development in the next earthly existence. For the undeveloped physical soul is entirely dominated by material nature and its impressions and has to work them out to a better advantage before it can rise in the scale of being.

A more developed humanity allows us to make a better and freer use of all the capacities and experiences that we derive from the vital and mental planes of being, to lean more for support upon these hidden planes, be less absorbed by the physical and to govern and modify the original nature of the physical being by greater vital forces and powers from the desire-world and greater and subtler mental forces and powers from the psychical and intellectual planes. By this development we are able to rise to higher altitudes of the intermediary existence between death and rebirth and to make a better and more rapid use of rebirth itself for a yet higher mental and spiritual development. But even so, in the physical being which still determines the greater part of our waking self, we act without definite consciousness of the worlds or planes which are the sources of our action. We are aware indeed of the life-plane and mind-plane of the physical being, but not of the life-plane and mind-plane proper or of the superior and larger vital and mental being which we are behind the veil of our ordinary consciousness. It is only at a high stage of development that we become aware of them and even then, ordinarily, only at the back of the action of our mentalised physical nature; we do not actually live on those planes, for if we did we could very soon arrive at the conscious control of the body by the life-power and of both by the sovereign mind; we should then be able to determine our physical and mental life to a very large extent by our will and knowledge as masters of our being and with a direct action of the mind on the life and body. By Yoga this power of transcending the physical self and taking possession of the higher selves may to a greater or less degree be acquired through a heightened and widened self-consciousness and self-mastery.

This may be done, on the side of Purusha, by drawing back from the physical self and its preoccupation with physical nature and through concentration of thought and will raising oneself into the vital and then into the mental self. By doing so we can become the vital being and draw up the physical self into that new consciousness so that we are only aware of the body, its nature and its actions as secondary circumstances of the Life-soul which we now are, used by it for its relations with the material world. A certain remoteness from physical being and then a superiority to it; a vivid sense of the body being a mere instrument or shell and easily detachable; an extraordinary effectivity of our desires on our physical being and life-environment; a great sense of power and ease in manipulating and directing the vital energy of which we now become vividly conscious, for its action is felt by us concretely, subtly physical in relation to the body, sensible in a sort of subtle density as an energy used by the mind; an awareness of the life-plane in us above the physical and knowledge and contact with the beings of the desire-world; a coming into action of new powers,—what are usually called occult powers or siddhis; a close sense of and sympathy with the Life-soul in the world and a knowledge or sensation of the emotions, desires, vital impulses of others; these are some of the signs of this new consciousness gained by Yoga.

But all this belongs to the inferior grades of spiritual experience and indeed is hardly more spiritual than the physical existence. We have in the same way to go yet higher and raise ourselves into the mental self. By doing so we can become the mental self and draw up the physical and vital being into it, so that life and body and their operations become to us minor circumstances of our being used by the Mind-soul which we now are for the execution of its lower purposes that belong to the material existence. Here too we acquire at first a certain remoteness from the life and the body and our real life seems to be on quite another plane than material man's, in contact with a subtler existence, a greater light of knowledge than the terrestrial, a far rarer and yet more sovereign energy; we are in touch in fact with the mental plane, aware of the mental worlds, can be in communication with its beings and powers. From that plane we behold the desire-world and the material existence as if below us, things that we can cast away from us if we will and in fact easily reject when we relinquish the body, so as to dwell in the mental or psychical heavens. But we can also, instead of being thus remote and detached, become rather superior to the life and body and the vital and material planes and act upon them with mastery from our new height of being. Another sort of dynamis than physical or vital energy, something that we may call pure mind-power and soul-force, which the developed human being uses indeed but derivatively and imperfectly, but which we can now use freely and with knowledge, becomes the ordinary process of our action, while desire-force and physical action fall into a secondary place and are only used with this new energy behind them and as its occasional channels. We are in touch and sympathy also with the Mind in cosmos, conscious of it, aware of the intentions, directions, thought-forces, struggle of subtle powers behind all happenings, which the ordinary man is ignorant of or can only obscurely infer from the physical happening, but which we can now see and feel directly before there is any physical sign or even vital intimation of their working. We acquire too the knowledge and sense of the mind-action of other beings whether on the physical plane or on those above it; and the higher capacities of the mental being,—occult powers or siddhis, but of a much rarer or subtler kind than those proper to the vital plane,—naturally awake in our consciousness.

All these however are circumstances of the lower triple world of our being, the *trailokya* of the ancient sages. Living on these we are, whatever the enlargement of our powers and our consciousness, still living within the limits of the cosmic gods and subject, though with a much subtler, easier and modified subjection, to the reign of Prakriti over Purusha. To achieve real freedom and mastery we have to ascend to a yet higher level of the many-plateaued mountain of our being.

# THE LADDER OF SELF-TRANSCENDENCE

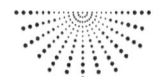

THE TRANSCENDENCE of this lower triple being and this lower triple world, to which ordinarily our consciousness and its powers and results are limited,—a transcendence described by the Vedic seers as an exceeding or breaking beyond the two firmaments of heaven and earth,—opens out a hierarchy of infinitudes to which the normal existence of man even in its highest and widest flights is still a stranger. Into that altitude, even to the lowest step of its hierarchy, it is difficult for him to rise. A separation, acute in practice though unreal in essence, divides the total being of man, the microcosm, as it divides also the world-being, the macrocosm. Both have a higher and a lower hemisphere, the *parārdha* and *aparārdha* of the ancient wisdom. The higher hemisphere is the perfect and eternal reign of the Spirit; for there it manifests without cessation or diminution its infinities, deploys the unconcealed glories of its illimitable existence, its illimitable consciousness and knowledge, its illimitable force and power, its illimitable beatitude. The lower hemisphere belongs equally to the Spirit; but here it is veiled, closely, thickly, by its inferior self-expression of limiting mind, confined life and dividing body. The Self in the lower hemisphere is shrouded in name and form; its consciousness is broken up by the division between the internal and external, the individual and universal; its vision and sense are turned outward; its force, limited by division of its consciousness, works in fetters; its knowledge, will, power, delight, divided by this division, limited by this limitation, are open to the experience of their contrary or perverse forms, to ignorance, weakness and suffering. We can indeed become aware of the true Self or Spirit in ourselves by turning our sense and vision inward; we can discover too the same Self or Spirit in the external world and its phenomena by plunging them there also inward through the veil of names and forms to that which dwells in these or else stands behind them. Our normal consciousness through this inward look may become by reflection aware of the infinite being, consciousness and delight of the Self and share in its passive or static infinity of these things. But we can only to a very limited extent share in its active or dynamic manifestation of knowledge, power and joy. Even this static identity by reflection cannot, ordinarily, be effected without a long and difficult effort and as the result of many lives of progressive self-development; for very firmly is our normal consciousness bound to the law of its lower hemisphere of being. To understand the possibility of transcending it at all, we must restate in a practical formula the relations of the worlds which constitute the two hemispheres.

All is determined by the Spirit, for all from subtlest existence to grossest matter is manifestation of the Spirit. But the Spirit, Self or Being determines the world it lives in and the experiences of its consciousness, force and delight in that world by some poise—among many possible—of the relations of Purusha and Prakriti, Soul and Nature,—some basic poise in one or other of its own cosmic principles. Poised in the principle of Matter, it becomes the physical self of a physical universe in the reign of a physical Nature. Spirit is then absorbed in its experience of Matter; it is dominated by the ignorance and inertia of the tamasic Power proper to physical existence. In the individual it becomes a materialised soul, *annamaya puruṣa*, whose life and mind have developed out of the ignorance and inertia of the material principle and are subject to their fundamental limitations. For life in Matter works in dependence on the body; mind in Matter works in dependence on the body and on the vital or nervous being; spirit itself in Matter is limited and divided in its self-relation and its powers by the limitations and divisions of this matter-governed and life-driven mind. This materialised soul lives bound to the physical body and its narrow superficial external consciousness, and it takes normally the experiences of its physical organs, its senses, its matter-bound life and mind, with at most some limited spiritual glimpses, as the whole truth of existence.

Man is a spirit, but a spirit that lives as a mental being in physical Nature; he is to his own self-consciousness a mind in a physical body. But at first he is this mental being materialised and he takes the materialised soul, *annamaya puruṣa*, for his real self. He is obliged to accept, as the Upanishad expresses it, Matter for the Brahman because his vision here sees Matter as that from which all is born, by which all lives and to which all return in their passing. His natural highest concept of Spirit is an Infinite, preferably an inconscient Infinite, inhabiting or pervading the material universe (which alone it really knows), and manifesting by the power of its presence all these forms around him. His natural highest conception of himself is a vaguely conceived soul or spirit, a soul manifested only by the physical life's experiences, bound up with physical phenomena and forced on its dissolution to return by an automatic necessity to the vast indeterminateness of the Infinite. But because he has the power of self-development, he can rise beyond these natural conceptions of the materialised soul; he can supplement them with a certain derivative experience drawn from supraphysical planes and worlds. He can concentrate in mind and develop the mental part of his being, usually at the expense of the fullness of his vital and physical life and in the end the mind predominates and can open to the Beyond. He can concentrate this self-liberating mind on the Spirit. Here too usually in the process he turns away more and more from his full mental and physical life; he limits or discourages their possibilities as much as his material foundation in nature will allow him. In the end his spiritual life predominates, destroys his earthward tendency and breaks its ties and limitations. Spiritualised, he places his real existence beyond in other worlds, in the heavens of the vital or mental plane; he begins to regard life on earth as a painful or troublesome incident or passage in which he can never arrive at any full enjoyment of his inner ideal self, his spiritual essence. Moreover, his highest conception of the Self or Spirit is apt to be more or less quietistic; for, as we have seen, it is its static infinity alone that he can entirely experience, the still freedom of Purusha unlimited by Prakriti, the Soul standing back from Nature. There may come indeed some divine dynamic manifestation in him, but it cannot rise entirely above the heavy limitations of physical Nature. The peace of the silent and passive Self is more easily attainable and he can more easily and fully hold it; too difficult for him is the bliss of an infinite activity, the dynamis of an immeasurable Power.

But the Spirit can be poised in the principle of Life, not in Matter. The

Spirit so founded becomes the vital self of a vital world, the Life-soul of a Life-energy in the reign of a consciously dynamic Nature. Absorbed in the experiences of the power and play of a conscious Life, it is dominated by the desire, activity and passion of the rajasic principle proper to vital existence. In the individual this spirit becomes a vital soul, *prāṇamaya puruṣa*, in whose nature the life-energies tyrannise over the mental and physical principles. The physical element in a vital world readily shapes its activities and formations in response to desire and its imaginations, it serves and obeys the passion and power of life and their formations and does not thwart or limit them as it does here on earth where life is a precarious incident in inanimate Matter. The mental element too is moulded and limited by the life-power, obeys it and helps only to enrich and fulfil the urge of its desires and the energy of its impulses. This vital soul lives in a vital body composed of a substance much subtler than physical matter; it is a substance surcharged with conscious energy, capable of much more powerful perceptions, capacities, sense-activities than any that the gross atomic elements of earth-matter can offer. Man too has in himself behind his physical being, subliminal to it, unseen and unknown, but very close to it and forming with it the most naturally active part of his existence, this vital soul, this vital nature and this vital body; a whole vital plane connected with the life-world or desire-world is hidden in us, a secret consciousness in which life and desire find their untrammelled play and their easy self-expression and from there throw their influences and formations on our outer life.

In proportion as the power of this vital plane manifests itself in man and takes hold of his physical being, this son of earth becomes a vehicle of the life energy, forceful in his desires, vehement in his passions and emotions, intensely dynamic in his action, more and more the rajasic man. It is possible now for him to awaken in his consciousness to the vital plane and to become the vital soul, *prāṇamaya puruṣa*, put on the vital nature and live in the secret vital as well as the visible physical body. If he achieves this change with some fullness or one-pointedness— usually it is under great and salutary limitations or attended by saving complexities—and without rising beyond these things, without climbing to a supra-vital height from which they can be used, purified, uplifted, he becomes the lower type of Asura or Titan, a Rakshasa in nature, a soul of sheer power and life-energy, magnified or racked by a force of unlimited desire and passion, hunted and driven by an active capacity and colossal rajasic ego, but in possession of far greater and more various powers than those of the physical man in the ordinary more inert earth-nature. Even if he develops mind greatly on the vital plane and uses its dynamic energy for self-control as well as for self-satisfaction, it will still be with an Asuric energism (*tapasyā*) although of a higher type and directed to a more governed satisfaction of the rajasic ego.

But for the vital plane also it is possible, even as on the physical, to rise to a certain spiritual greatness in its own kind. It is open to the vital man to lift himself beyond the conceptions and energies natural to the desire-soul and the desire-plane. He can develop a higher mentality and, within the conditions of the vital being, concentrate upon some realisation of the Spirit or Self behind or beyond its forms and powers. In this spiritual realisation there would be a less strong necessity of quietism; for there would be a greater possibility of an active effectuation of the bliss and power of the Eternal, mightier and more self-satisfied powers, a richer flowering of the dynamic Infinite. Nevertheless that effectuality could never come anywhere near to a true and integral perfection; for the conditions of the desire-world are like those of the physical improper to the development of the complete spiritual life. The vital being too must develop spirit to the detriment of his fullness, activity and force of life in the lower hemisphere of our existence and turn in the end away from the vital formula, away from life either to the Silence or to an ineffable Power beyond him. If he does not withdraw from life, he must remain enchained by life, limited in his self-fulfilment by the downward pull of the desire-world and its dominant rajasic principle. On the vital plane also, in its own right alone, a perfect perfection is impossible; the soul that attains only so far would have to return to the physical life for a greater experience, a higher self-development, a more direct ascent to the Spirit.

Above matter and life stands the principle of mind, nearer to the secret Origin of things. The Spirit poised in mind becomes the mental self of a mental world and dwells there in the reign of its own pure and luminous mental Nature. There it acts in the intrinsic freedom of the cosmic Intelligence supported by the combined workings of a psycho-mental and a higher emotional mind-force, subtilised and enlightened by the clarity and happiness of the sattwic principle proper to the mental existence. In the individual the spirit so poised becomes a mental soul, *manomaya puruṣa*, in whose nature the clarity and luminous power of the mind acts in its own right independent of any limitation or oppression by the vital or corporeal instruments; it rather rules and determines entirely the forms of its body and the powers of its life. For mind in its own plane is not limited by life and obstructed by matter as it is here in the earth-process. This mental soul lives in a mental or subtle body which enjoys capacities of knowledge, perception, sympathy and interpenetration with other beings hardly imaginable by us and a free, delicate and extensive mentalised sense-faculty not limited by the grosser conditions of the life nature or the physical nature.

Man too has in himself, subliminal, unknown and unseen, concealed behind his waking consciousness and visible organism this mental soul, mental nature, mental body and a mental plane, not materialised, in which the principle of Mind is at home and not as here at strife with a world which is alien to it, obstructive to its freedom and corruptive of its purity and clearness. All the higher faculties of man, his intellectual and psycho-mental being and powers, his higher emotional life awaken and increase in proportion as this mental plane in him presses upon him. For the more it manifests, the more it influences the physical parts, the more it enriches and elevates the corresponding mental plane of the embodied nature. At a certain pitch of its increasing sovereignty it can make man truly man and not merely a reasoning animal; for it gives then its characteristic force to that mental being within us which our humanity is in the inwardly governing but still too hampered essence of its psychological structure.

It is possible for man to awaken to this higher mental consciousness, to become this mental being,[1] put on this mental nature and live not only in the vital and physical sheaths, but in this mental body. If there were a sufficient completeness in this transformation he would become capable of a life and a being at least half divine. For he would enjoy powers and a vision and perceptions beyond the scope of this ordinary life and body; he would govern all by the clarities of pure knowledge; he would be united to other beings by a sympathy of love and happiness; his emotions would be lifted to the perfection of the psycho-mental plane, his sensations rescued from grossness, his intellect subtle, pure and flexible, delivered from the deviations of the impure pranic energy and the obstructions of matter. And he would develop too the reflection of a wisdom and bliss higher than any mental joy and knowledge; for he could receive more fully and without our incompetent mind's deforming and falsifying mixture the inspirations and intuitions that are the arrows of the supramental Light and form his perfected mental existence in the mould and power of that vaster splendour. He could then realise too the self or Spirit in a much larger and more luminous and more intimate intensity than is now possible and with a greater play of its active power and bliss in the satisfied harmony of his existence.

And to our ordinary notions this may well seem to be a consummate perfection, something to which man might aspire in his highest flights of idealism. No doubt, it would be a sufficient perfection for the pure mental being in its own character; but it would still fall far below the greater possibilities of the spiritual nature. For here too our spiritual realisation would be subject to the limitations of the mind which is in the nature of a reflected, diluted and diffused or a narrowly intensive light, not the vast and comprehensive self-existent luminosity and joy of the Spirit. That vaster light, that profounder bliss are beyond the mental reaches. Mind indeed can never be a perfect instrument of the Spirit; a supreme self-expression is not possible in its movements because to separate, divide, limit is its very character. Even if mind could be free from all positive falsehood and error, even if it could be all intuitive and infallibly intuitive, it could still present and organise only half-truths or separate truths and these too not in their own body but in luminous representative figures put together to make an accumulated total or a massed structure. Therefore the self-perfecting mental being here must either depart into pure spirit by the shedding of its lower existence or return upon the physical life to develop in it a capacity not yet found in our mental and psychic nature. This is what the Upanishad expresses when it says that the heavens attained by the mind Purusha are those to which man is lifted by the rays of the sun, the diffused, separated, though intense beams of the supramental truth-consciousness, and from these it has to return to the earthly existence. But the illuminates who renouncing earth-life go beyond through the gateways of the sun, do not return hither. The mental being exceeding his sphere does not return because by that transition he enters a high range of existence peculiar to the superior hemisphere. He cannot bring down its greater spiritual nature into this lower triplicity; for here the mental being is the highest expression of the Self. Here the triple mental, vital and physical body provides almost the whole range of our capacity and cannot suffice for that greater consciousness; the vessel has not been built to contain a greater godhead or to house the splendours of this supramental force and knowledge.

This limitation is true only so long as man remains closed within the boundaries of the mental Maya. If he rises into the knowledge-self beyond the highest mental stature, if he becomes the knowledge-soul, the Spirit poised in gnosis, *vijñānamaya puruṣa*, and puts on the nature of its infinite truth and power, if he lives in the knowledge-sheath, the causal body as well as in these subtle mental, interlinking vital and grosser physical sheaths or bodies, then, but then only he will be able to draw down entirely into his terrestrial existence the fullness of the infinite spiritual consciousness; only then will he avail to raise his total being and even his whole manifested, embodied expressive nature into the spiritual kingdom. But this is difficult in the extreme; for the causal body opens itself readily to the consciousness and capacities of the spiritual planes and belongs in its nature to the higher hemisphere of existence, but it is either not developed at all in man or only as yet crudely developed and organised and veiled behind many intervening portals of the subliminal in us. It draws its stuff from the plane of the truth-knowledge and the plane of the infinite bliss and these pertain altogether to a still inaccessible higher hemisphere. Shedding upon this lower existence their truth and light and joy they are the source of all that we call spirituality and all that we call perfection. But this infiltration comes from behind thick coverings through which they arrive so tempered and weakened that they are entirely obscured in the materiality of our physical perceptions, grossly distorted and perverted in our vital impulses, perverted too though a little less grossly in our ideative seekings, minimised even in the comparative purity and intensity of the highest intuitive ranges of our mental nature. The supramental principle is secretly lodged in all existence. It is there even in the grossest materiality, it preserves and governs the lower worlds by its hidden power and law; but that power veils itself and that law works unseen through the shackled limitations and limping deformations of the lesser rule of our physical, vital, mental Nature. Yet its governing presence in the lowest forms assures us, because of the unity of all existence, that there is a possibility of their awakening, a possibility even of their perfect manifestation here in spite of every veil, in spite of all the mass of our apparent disabilities, in spite of the incapacity or unwillingness of our mind and life and body. And what is possible, must one day be, for that is the law of the omnipotent Spirit.

The character of these higher states of the soul and their greater worlds of spiritual Nature is necessarily difficult to seize. Even the Upanishads and the Veda only shadow them out by figures, hints and symbols. Yet it is necessary to attempt some account of their principles and practical effect so far as they can be grasped by the mind that stands on the border of the two hemispheres. The passage beyond that border would be the culmination, the completeness of the Yoga of self-transcendence by self-knowledge. The soul that aspires to perfection, draws back and upward, says the Upanishad, from the physical into the vital and from the vital into the mental Purusha, from the mental into the knowledge-soul and from that self of knowledge into the bliss Purusha. This self of bliss is the conscious foundation of perfect Sachchidananda and to pass into it completes the soul's ascension. The mind therefore must try to give to itself some account of this decisive transformation of the embodied consciousness, this radiant transfiguration and self-exceeding of our ever aspiring nature. The description mind can arrive at, can never be adequate to the thing itself, but it may point at least to some indicative shadow of it or perhaps some half-luminous image.

---

1. I include here in mind, not only the highest range of mind ordinarily known to man, but yet higher ranges to which he has either no current faculty of admission or else only a partial and mixed reception of some faint portion of their powers,—the illumined mind, the intuition and finally the creative Overmind or Maya which stands far above and is the source of our present existence. If mind is to be understood only as Reason or human intelligence, then the free mental being and its state would be something much more limited and very inferior to the description given here.

# VIJNANA OR GNOSIS

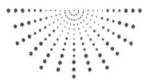

IN OUR perfect self-transcendence we pass out and up from the ignorance or half-enlightenment of our mental conscious-being into a greater wisdom-self and truth-power above it, there to dwell in the unwalled light of a divine knowledge. The mental man that we are is changed into the gnostic soul, the truth-conscious godhead, the *vijñāna-maya* Purusha. Seated on that level of the hill of our ascension we are in a quite different plane from this material, this vital, this mental poise of the universal spirit, and with this change changes too all our view and experience of our soul-life and of the world around us. We are born into a new soul-status and put on a new nature; for according to the status of the soul is the status of the Prakriti. At each transition of the world-ascent, from matter to life, from life to mind, from mind bound to free intelligence, as the latent, half-manifested or already manifest soul rises to a higher and higher level of being, the nature also is elevated into a superior working, a wider consciousness, a vaster force and an intenser or larger range and joy of existence. But the transition from the mind-self to the knowledge-self is the great and the decisive transition in the Yoga. It is the shaking off of the last hold on us of the cosmic ignorance and our firm foundation in the Truth of things, in a consciousness infinite and eternal and inviolable by obscurity, falsehood, suffering or error.

This is the first summit which enters into the divine perfection, *sādharmya*, *sādṛśya*; for all the rest only look up to it or catch some rays of its significance. The highest heights of mind or of overmind come still within the belt of a mitigated ignorance; they can refract a divine Light but not pass it on in undiminished power to our lower members. For so long as we are within the triple stratum of mind, life and body, our active nature continues to work in the force of the ignorance even when the soul in Mind possesses something of the knowledge. And even if the soul were to reflect or to represent all the largeness of the knowledge in its mental consciousness, it would be unable to mobilise it rightly in force of action. The truth in its action might greatly increase, but it would still be pursued by a limitation, still condemned to a divisibility which would prevent it from working integrally in the power of the infinite. The power of a divinely illumined mind may be immense compared with ordinary powers, but it will still be subject to incapacity and there can be no perfect correspondence between the force of the effective will and the light of the idea which inspires it. The infinite Presence may be there in status, but the dynamis of the operations of nature still belongs to the lower Prakriti, must follow its triple modes of working and cannot give any adequate form to the greatness within it. This is the tragedy of ineffectivity, of the hiatus between ideal and effective will, of our constant incapacity to work out in living form and action the truth we feel in our inner consciousness that pursues all the aspiration of mind and life towards the divinity behind them. But the *vijñāna* or gnosis is not only truth but truth power, it is the very working of the infinite and divine nature; it is the divine knowledge one with the divine will in the force and delight of a spontaneous and luminous and inevitable self-fulfilment. By the gnosis, then, we change our human into a divine nature.

What then is this gnosis and how can we describe it? Two opposite errors have to be avoided, two misconceptions that disfigure opposite sides of the truth of gnosis. One error of intellect-bounded thinkers takes *vijñāna* as synonymous with the other Indian term *buddhi* and *buddhi* as synonymous with the reason, the discerning intellect, the logical intelligence. The systems that accept this significance, pass at once from a plane of pure intellect to a plane of pure spirit. No intermediate power is recognised, no diviner action of knowledge than the pure reason is admitted; the limited human means for fixing truth is taken for the highest possible dynamics of consciousness, its topmost force and original movement. An opposite error, a misconception of the mystics identifies *vijñāna* with the consciousness of the Infinite free from all ideation or else ideation packed into one essence of thought, lost to other dynamic action in the single and invariable idea of the One. This is the *caitanyaghana* of the Upanishad and is one movement or rather one thread of the many-aspected movement of the gnosis. The gnosis, the Vijnana, is not only this concentrated consciousness of the infinite Essence; it is also and at the same time an infinite knowledge of the myriad play of the Infinite. It contains all ideation (not mental but supramental), but it is not limited by ideation, for it far exceeds all ideative movement. Nor is the gnostic ideation in its character an intellectual thinking; it is not what we call the reason, not a concentrated intelligence. For the reason is mental in its methods, mental in its acquisitions, mental in its basis, but the ideative method of the gnosis is self-luminous, supramental, its yield of thought-light spontaneous, not proceeding by acquisition, its thought-basis a rendering of conscious identities, not a translation of the impressions born of indirect contacts. There is a relation and even a sort of broken identity between the two forms of thought; for one proceeds covertly from the other, mind is born from that which is beyond mind. But they act on different planes and reverse each other's process.

Even the purest reason, the most luminous rational intellectuality is not the gnosis. Reason or intellect is only the lower *buddhi*; it is dependent for its action on the percepts of the sense-mind and on the concepts of the mental intelligence. It is not like the gnosis, self-luminous, authentic, making the subject one with the object. There is, indeed, a higher form of the *buddhi* that can be called the intuitive mind or intuitive reason, and this by its intuitions, its inspirations, its swift revelatory vision, its luminous insight and discrimination can do the work of the reason with a higher power, a swifter action, a greater and spontaneous certitude. It acts in a self-light of the truth which does not depend upon the torch-flares of the sense-mind and its limited uncertain percepts; it proceeds not by intelligent but by visional concepts: it is a kind of truth-vision, truth-hearing, truth-memory, direct truth-discernment. This true and authentic intuition must be distinguished from a power of the ordinary mental reason which is too easily confused with it, the power of involved reasoning that reaches its conclusion by a bound and does not need the ordinary steps of the logical mind. The logical reason proceeds pace after pace and tries the sureness of each step like a man who is walking over unsafe ground and has to test by the hesitating touch of his foot each span of soil that he perceives with his eye. But this other supralogical process of the reason is a motion of rapid insight or swift discernment; it proceeds by a stride or leap, like a man who springs from one sure spot to another point of sure footing,—or at least held by him to be sure. He sees the space he covers in one compact and flashing view, but he does not distinguish or measure either by eye or touch its successions, features and circumstances. This movement has something of the sense of power of the intuition, something of its velocity, some appearance of its light and certainty, and we always are apt to take it for the intuition. But our assumption is an error and, if we trust to it, may lead us into grievous blunders.

It is even thought by the intellectualists that the intuition itself is nothing more than this rapid process in which the whole action of the logical mind is swiftly done or perhaps half-consciously or subconsciously done, not deliberately worked out in its reasoned method. In its nature, however, this proceeding is quite different from the intuition and it is not necessarily a truth-movement. The power of its leap may end in a stumble, its swiftness may betray, its certainty is too often a confident error. The validity of its conclusions must always depend on a subsequent verification or support from the evidence of the sense-perceptions or a rational linking of intelligent conceptions must intervene to explain to it its own certitudes. This lower light may indeed receive very readily a mixture of actual intuition into it and then a pseudo-intuitive or half-intuitive mind is created, very misleading by its frequent luminous successes palliating a whirl of intensely self-assured false certitudes. The true intuition on the contrary carries in itself its own guarantee of truth; it is sure and infallible within its limits. And so long as it is pure intuition and does not admit into itself any mixture of sense-error or intellectual ideation, it is never contradicted by experience: the intuition may be verified by the reason or the sense-perception afterwards, but its truth does not depend on that verification, it is assured by an automatic self-evidence. If the reason depending on its inferences contradicts the greater light, it will be found in the end on ampler knowledge that the intuitional conclusion was correct and that the more plausible rational and inferential conclusion was an error. For the true intuition proceeds from the self-existent truth of things and is secured by that self-existent truth and not by any indirect, derivatory or dependent method of arriving at knowledge.

But even the intuitive reason is not the gnosis; it is only an edge of light of the supermind finding its way by flashes of illumination into the mentality like lightnings in dim and cloudy places. Its inspirations, revelations, intuitions, self-luminous discernings are messages from a higher knowledge-plane that make their way opportunely into our lower level of consciousness. The very character of the intuitive mind sets a gulf of great difference between its action and the action of the self-contained gnosis. In the first place it acts by separate and limited illuminations and its truth is restricted to the often narrow reach or the one brief spot of knowledge lit up by that one lightning-flash with which its intervention begins and terminates. We see the action of the instinct in animals,—an automatic intuition in that vital or sense-mind which is the highest and surest instrument that the animal has to rely on, since it does not possess the human light of the reason, only a cruder and yet ill-formed intelligence. And we can observe at once that the marvellous truth of this instinct which seems so much surer than the reason, is limited in the bird, beast or insect to some particular and restricted utility it is admitted to serve. When the vital mind of the animal tries to act beyond that restricted limit, it blunders in a much blinder way than the reason of man and has to learn with difficulty by a succession of sense-experiences. The higher mental intuition of the human being is an inner visional, not a sense intuition; for it illumines the intelligence and not the sense-mind, it is self-conscious and luminous, not a half-subconscious blind light: it is freely self-acting, not mechanically automatic. But still, even when it is not marred by the imitative pseudo-intuition, it is restricted in man like the instinct in the animal, restricted to a particular purpose of will or knowledge as is the instinct to a particular life utility or Nature purpose. And when the intelligence, as is its almost invariable habit, tries to make use of it, to apply it, to add to it, it builds round the intuitive nucleus in its own characteristic fashion a mass of mixed truth and error. More often than not, by foisting an element of sense-error and conceptual error into the very substance of the intuition or by coating it up in mental additions and deviations, it not merely deflects but deforms its truth and converts it into a falsehood. At the best therefore the intuition gives us only a limited, though an intense light; at the worst, through our misuse of it or false imitations of it, it may lead us into perplexities and confusions which the less ambitious intellectual reason avoids by remaining satisfied with its own safe and plodding method,—safe for the inferior purposes of the reason, though never a satisfying guide to the inner truth of things.

It is possible to cultivate and extend the use of the intuitive mind in proportion as we rely less predominantly upon the reasoning intelligence. We may train our mentality not to seize, as it does now, upon every separate flash of intuitive illumination for its own inferior purposes, not to precipitate our thought at once into a crystallising intellectual action around it; we can train it to think in a stream of successive and connected intuitions, to pour light upon light in a brilliant and triumphant series. We shall succeed in this difficult change in proportion as we purify the interfering intelligence,—if we can reduce in it the element of material thought enslaved to the external appearances of things, the element of vital thought enslaved to the wishes, desires, impulses of the lower nature, the element of intellectual thought enslaved to our preferred, already settled or congenial ideas, conceptions, opinions, fixed operations of intelligence, if, having reduced to a minimum those elements, we can replace them by an intuitive vision and sense of things, an intuitive insight into appearances, an intuitive will, an intuitive ideation. This is hard enough for our consciousness naturally bound by the triple tie of mentality, vitality, corporeality to its own imperfection and ignorance, the upper, middle and lower cord in the Vedic parable of the soul's bondage, cords of the mixed truth and falsehood of appearances by which Shunahshepa was bound to the post of sacrifice.

But even if this difficult thing were perfectly accomplished, still the intuition would not be the gnosis; it would only be its thin prolongation into mind or its sharp edge of first entrance. The difference, not easy to define except by symbols, may be expressed if we take the Vedic image in which the Sun represents the gnosis and the sky, mid-air and earth the mentality, vitality, physicality of man and of the universe. Living on the earth, climbing into the mid-air or even winging in the sky, the mental being, the *manomaya* Purusha, would still live in the rays of the sun and not in its bodily light. And in those rays he would see things not as they are, but as reflected in his organ of vision, deformed by its faults or limited in their truth by its restrictions. But the *vijñānamaya* Purusha lives in the Sun itself, in the very body and blaze of the true light;[1] he knows this light to be his own self-luminous being and he sees besides all that dwells in the rays of the sun, sees the whole truth of the lower triplicity and each thing that is in it. He sees it not by reflection in a mental organ of vision, but with the Sun of gnosis itself as his eye,—for the Sun, says the Veda, is the eye of the gods. The mental being, even in the intuitive mind, can perceive the truth only by a brilliant reflection or limited communication and subject to the restrictions and the inferior capacity of the mental vision; but the supramental being sees it by the gnosis itself, from the very centre and outwelling fount of the truth, in its very form and by its own spontaneous and self-illumining process. For the Vijnana is a direct and divine as opposed to an indirect and human knowledge.

The nature of the gnosis can only be indicated to the intellect by contrasting it with the nature of the intellect, and even then the phrases we must use cannot illuminate unless aided by some amount of actual experience. For what language forged by the reason can express the suprarational? Fundamentally, this is the difference between these two powers that the mental reason proceeds with labour from ignorance to truth, but the gnosis has in itself the direct contact, the immediate vision, the easy and constant possession of the truth and has no need of seeking or any kind of procedure. The reason starts with appearances and labours, never or seldom losing at least a partial dependence on appearances, to arrive at the truth behind them; it shows the truth in the light of the appearances. The gnosis starts from the truth and shows the appearances in the light of the truth; it is itself the body of the truth and its spirit. The reason proceeds by inference, it concludes; but the gnosis proceeds by identity or vision,—it is, sees and knows. As directly as the physical vision sees and grasps the appearance of objects, so and far more directly the gnosis sees and grasps the truth of things. But where the physical sense gets into relation with objects by a veiled contact, the gnosis gets into identity with things by an unveiled oneness. Thus it is able to know all things as a man knows his own existence, simply, convincingly, directly. To the reason only what the senses give is direct knowledge, *pratyakṣa*, the rest of truth is arrived at indirectly; to the gnosis all its truth is direct knowledge, *pratyakṣa*. Therefore the truth gained by the intellect is an acquisition over which there hangs always a certain shadow of doubt, an incompleteness, a surrounding penumbra of night and ignorance or half-knowledge, a possibility of alteration or annullation by farther knowledge. The truth of the gnosis is free from doubt, self-evident, self-existent, irrefragable, absolute.

The reason has as its first instrument observation general, analytical and synthetic; it aids itself by comparison, contrast and analogy,—proceeds from experience to indirect knowledge by logical processes of deduction, induction, all kinds of inference,—rests upon memory, reaches out beyond itself by imagination, secures itself by judgment: all is a process of groping and seeking. The gnosis does not seek, it possesses. Or if it has to enlighten, it does not even then seek; it reveals, it illumines. In a consciousness transmuted from intelligence to gnosis, imagination would be replaced by truth-inspiration, mental judgment would give place to a self-luminous discerning. The slow and stumbling logical process from reasoning to conclusion would be pushed out by a swift intuitive proceeding; the conclusion or fact would be seen at once in its own right, by its own self-sufficient witness, and all the evidence by which we arrive at it would be seen too at once, along with it, in the same comprehensive figure, not as its evidence, but as its intimate conditions, connections and relations, its constituent parts or its wings of circumstance. Mental and sense observation would be changed into an inner vision using the instruments as channels, but not dependent on them as the mind in us is blind and deaf without the physical senses, and this vision would see not merely the thing, but all its truth, its forces, powers, the eternities within it. Our uncertain memory would fall away and there would come in its place a luminous possession of knowledge, the divine memory that is not a store of acquisition, but holds all things always contained in the consciousness, a memory at once of past, present and future.

For while the reason proceeds from moment to moment of time and loses and acquires and again loses and again acquires, the gnosis dominates time in a one view and perpetual power and links past, present and future in their indivisible connections, in a single continuous map of knowledge, side by side. The gnosis starts from the totality which it immediately possesses; it sees parts, groups and details only in relation to the totality and in one vision with it: the mental reason cannot really see the totality at all and does not know fully any whole except by starting from an analysis and synthesis of its parts, masses and details; otherwise its whole-view is always a vague apprehension or an imperfect comprehension or a confused summary of indistinct features. The reason deals with constituents and processes and properties; it tries in vain to form by them an idea of the thing in itself, its reality, its essence. But the gnosis sees the thing in itself first, penetrates to its original and eternal nature, adjoins its processes and properties only as a self-expression of its nature. The reason dwells in the diversity and is its prisoner: it deals with things separately and treats each as a separate existence, as it deals with sections of Time and divisions of Space; it sees unity only in a sum or by elimination of diversity or as a general conception and a vacant figure. But the gnosis dwells in the unity and knows by it all the nature of the diversities; it starts from the unity and sees diversities only of a unity, not diversities constituting the one, but a unity constituting its own multitudes. The gnostic knowledge, the gnostic sense does not recognise any real division; it does not treat things separately as if they were independent of their true and original oneness. The reason deals with the finite and is helpless before the infinite: it can conceive of it as an indefinite extension in which the finite acts, but the infinite in itself it can with difficulty conceive and cannot at all grasp or penetrate. But the gnosis is, sees and lives in the infinite; it starts always from the infinite and knows finite things only in their relation to the infinite and in the sense of the infinite.

If we would describe the gnosis as it is in its own awareness, not thus imperfectly as it is to us in contrast with our own reason and intelligence, it is hardly possible to speak of it except in figures and symbols. And first we must remember that the gnostic level, Mahat, Vijnana, is not the supreme plane of our consciousness, but a middle or link plane. Interposed between the triune glory of the utter Spirit, the infinite existence, consciousness and bliss of the Eternal and our lower triple being and nature, it is as if it stood there as the mediating, formulated, organising and creative wisdom, power and joy of the Eternal. In the gnosis Sachchidananda gathers up the light of his unseizable existence and pours it out on the soul in the shape and power of a divine knowledge, a divine will and a divine bliss of existence. It is as if infinite light were gathered up into the compact orb of the sun and lavished on all that depends upon the sun in radiances that continue for ever. But the gnosis is not only light, it is force; it is creative knowledge, it is the self-effective truth of the divine Idea. This idea is not creative imagination, not something that constructs in a void, but light and power of eternal substance, truth-light full of truth-force; and it brings out what is latent in being, it does not create a fiction that never was in being. The ideation of the gnosis is radiating light-stuff of the consciousness of the eternal Existence; each ray is a truth. The will in the gnosis is a conscious force of eternal knowledge; it throws the consciousness and substance of being into infallible forms of truth-power, forms that embody the idea and make it faultlessly effective, and it works out each truth-power and each truth-form spontaneously and rightly according to its nature. Because it carries this creative force of the divine Idea, the Sun, the lord and symbol of the gnosis, is described in the Veda as the Light which is the father of all things, Surya Savitri, the Wisdom-Luminous who is the bringer-out into manifest existence. This creation is inspired by the divine delight, the eternal Ananda; it is full of the joy of its own truth and power, it creates in bliss, creates out of bliss, creates that which is blissful. Therefore the world of the gnosis, the supramental world is the true and the happy creation, *ṛtam, bhadram,* since all in it shares in the perfect joy that made it. A divine radiance of undeviating knowledge, a divine power of unfaltering will and a divine ease of unstumbling bliss are the nature or Prakriti of the soul in supermind, in *vijñāna.*

The stuff of the gnostic or supramental plane is made of the perfect absolutes of all that is here imperfect and relative and its movement of the reconciled interlockings and happy fusions of all that here are opposites. For behind the appearance of these opposites are their truths and the truths of the Eternal are not in conflict with each other; our mind's and life's opposites transformed in the supermind into their own true spirit link together and are seen as tones and colourings of an eternal Reality and everlasting Ananda. Supermind or Gnosis is the supreme Truth, the supreme Thought, the supreme Word, the supreme Sight, the supreme Will-Idea; it is the inner and outer extension of the Infinite who is beyond Space, the unfettered Time of the Eternal who is timeless, the supernal harmony of all absolutes of the Absolute.

To the envisaging mind there are three powers of the Vijnana. Its supreme power knows and receives into it from above all the infinite existence, consciousness and bliss of the Ishwara; it is in its highest height the absolute knowledge and force of eternal Sachchidananda. Its second power concentrates the Infinite into a dense luminous consciousness, *caitanyaghana* or *cidghana,* the seed-state of the divine consciousness in which are contained living and concrete all the immutable principles of the divine being and all the inviolable truths of the divine conscious-idea and nature. Its third power brings or looses out these things by the effective ideation, vision, authentic identities of the divine knowledge, movement of the divine will-force, vibration of the divine delight intensities into a universal harmony, an illimitable diversity, a manifold rhythm of their powers, forms and interplay of living consequences. The mental Purusha rising into the *vijñānamaya* must ascend into these three powers. It must turn by conversion of its movements into the movements of the gnosis its mental perception, ideation, will, pleasure into radiances of the divine knowledge, pulsations of the divine will-force, waves and floods of the divine delight-seas. It must convert its conscious stuff of mental nature into the *cidghana* or dense self-luminous consciousness. It must transform its conscious substance into a gnostic self or Truth-self of infinite Sachchidananda. These three movements are described in the Isha Upanishad, the first as *vyūha*, the marshalling of the rays of the Sun of gnosis in the order of the Truth-consciousness, the second as *samū ha*, the gathering together of the rays into the body of the Sun of gnosis, the third as the vision of that Sun's fairest form of all in which the soul most intimately possesses its oneness with the infinite Purusha.[2] The Supreme above, in him, around, everywhere and the soul dwelling in the Supreme and one with it,—the infinite power and truth of the Divine concentrated in his own concentrated luminous soul nature,—a radiant activity of the divine knowledge, will and joy perfect in the natural action of the Prakriti,—this is the fundamental experience of the mental being transformed and fulfilled and sublimated in the perfection of the gnosis.

---

1. So the Sun is called in the Veda, *ṛtaṁ jyotiḥ*.
2. *Sūrya raśmīn vyūha samūha tejo yat te kalyāṇatamaṁ rūpaṁ tat te paśyāmi yo 'sāv asau puruṣaḥ so 'ham asmi*. The Veda describes the *vijñāna* plane as *ṛtaṁ satyaṁ bṛhat*, the Right, Truth , Vast, the same triple idea differently expressed . *ṛtam* is the action of the divine knowledge, will and joy in the lines of the truth, the play of the truth-consciousness. *Satyam* is the truth of being which so acts, the dynamic essence of the truth-consciousness. *Bṛhat* is the infinity of Sachchidananda out of which the other two proceed and in which they are founded.

# THE CONDITIONS OF ATTAINMENT TO THE GNOSIS

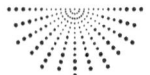

KNOWLEDGE is the first principle of the Vijnana, but knowledge is not its only power. The Truth-consciousness, like every other plane, founds itself upon that particular principle which is naturally the key of all its motions; but it is not limited by it, it contains all the other powers of existence. Only the character and working of these other powers is modified and moulded into conformity with its own original and dominant law; intelligence, life, body, will, consciousness, bliss are all luminous, awake, instinct with divine knowledge. This is indeed the process of Purusha-Prakriti everywhere; it is the key-movement of all the hierarchy and graded harmonies of manifested existence.

In the mental being mind-sense or intelligence is the original and dominant principle. The mental being in the mind-world where he is native is in his central and determining nature intelligence; he is a centre of intelligence, a massed movement of intelligence, a receptive and radiating action of intelligence. He has the intelligent sense of his own existence, the intelligent sense of other existence than his own, the intelligent sense of his own nature and activities and the activities of others, the intelligent sense of the nature of things and persons and their relations with himself and each other. That makes up his experience of existence. He has no other knowledge of existence, no knowledge of life and matter except as they make themselves sensible to him and capable of being seized by his mental intelligence; what he does not sense and conceive, is to him practically non-existent, or at least alien to his world and his nature.

Man is in his principle a mental being, but not one living in a mind world, but in a dominantly physical existence; his is a mind cased in Matter and conditioned by Matter. Therefore he has to start with the action of the physical senses which are all channels of material contact; he does not start with the mind-sense. But even so he does not and cannot make free use of anything conveyed by these physical organs until and unless they are taken hold of by the mind-sense and turned into stuff and value of his intelligent being. What is in the lower subhuman submental world a pranic, a nervous, a dynamic action and reaction that proceeds very well without any need of translation into mind-terms or government by mind, has in him to be raised and offered to some kind of intelligence. In order to be characteristically human it has to become first a sense of force, sense of desire, sense of will, sense of intelligent will-action or mentally conscious sense of force-action. His lower delight of being translates itself into a sense of mental or mentalised vital or physical pleasure and its perversion pain, or into a mental or mentalised feeling-sensation of liking and disliking, or into an intelligence of delight and failure of delight,—all phenomena of the intelligent mind-sense. So too that which is above him and that which is around him and in which he lives,—God, the universal being, the cosmic Forces,—are non-existent and unreal to him until his mind awakes to them and gets, not yet their true truth, but some idea, observation, inference, imagination of things supersensuous, some mental sense of the Infinite, some intelligent interpreting consciousness of the forces of the superself above and around him.

All changes when we pass from mind to gnosis; for there a direct inherent knowledge is the central principle. The gnostic (*vijñānamaya*) being is in its character a truth-consciousness, a centre and circumference of the truth-vision of things, a massed movement or subtle body of gnosis. Its action is a self-fulfilling and radiating action of the truth-power of things according to the inner law of their deepest truest self and nature. This truth of things at which we must arrive before we can enter into the gnosis,—for in that all exists and from that all originates on the gnostic plane,—is, first of all, a truth of unity, of oneness, but of unity originating diversity, unity in multiplicity and still unity always, an indefeasible oneness. State of gnosis, the condition of *vijñānamaya* being, is impossible without an ample and close self-identification of ourselves with all existence and with all existences, a universal pervasiveness, a universal comprehension or containing, a certain all-in-allness. The gnostic Purusha has normally the consciousness of itself as infinite, normally too the consciousness of containing the world in itself and exceeding it; it is not like the divided mental being normally bound to a consciousness that feels itself contained in the world and a part of it. It follows that a deliverance from the limiting and imprisoning ego is the first elementary step towards the being of the gnosis; for so long as we live in the ego, it is idle to hope for this higher reality, this vast self-consciousness, this true self-knowledge. The least reversion to ego-thought, ego-action, ego-will brings back the consciousness tumbling out of such gnostic Truth as it has attained into the falsehoods of the divided mind-nature. A secure universality of being is the very basis of this luminous higher consciousness. Abandoning all rigid separateness (but getting instead a certain transcendent overlook or independence) we have to feel ourselves one with all things and beings, to identify ourselves with them, to become aware of them as ourselves, to feel their being as our own, to admit their consciousness as part of ours, to contact their energy as intimate to our energy, to learn how to be one self with all. That oneness is not indeed all that is needed, but it is a first condition and without it there is no gnosis.

This universality is impossible to achieve in its completeness so long as we continue to feel ourselves, as we now feel, a consciousness lodged in an individual mind, life and body. There has to be a certain elevation of the Purusha out of the physical and even out of the mental into the *vijñānamaya* body. No longer can the brain nor its corresponding mental "lotus" remain the centre of our thinking, no longer the heart nor its corresponding "lotus" the originating centre of our emotional and sensational being. The conscious centre of our being, our thought, our will and action, even the original force of our sensations and emotions rise out of the body and mind and take a free station above them. No longer have we the sensation of living in the body, but are above it as its lord, possessor or Ishwara and at the same time encompass it with a wider consciousness than that of the imprisoned physical sense. Now we come to realise with a very living force of reality, normal and continuous, what the sages meant when they spoke of the soul carrying the body or when they said that the soul is not in the body, but the body in the soul. It is from above the body and not from the brain that we shall ideate and will; the brain-action will become only a response and movement of the physical machinery to the shock of the thought-force and will-force from above. All will be originated from above; from above, all that corresponds in gnosis to our present mental activity takes place.[1]

But this centre and this action are free, not bound, not dependent on the physical machine, not clamped to a narrow ego-sense. It is not involved in body; it is not shut up in a separated individuality feeling out for clumsy contacts with the world outside or groping inward for its own deeper spirit. For in this great transformation we begin to have a consciousness not shut up in a generating box, but diffused freely and extending self-existently everywhere; there is or may be a centre, but it is a convenience for individual action, not rigid, not constitutive or separative. The very nature of our conscious activities is henceforth universal; one with those of the universal being, it proceeds from universality to a supple and variable individualisation. It has become the awareness of an infinite being who acts always universally though with emphasis on an individual formation of its energies. But this emphasis is differential rather than separative, and this formation is no longer what we now understand by individuality; there is no longer a petty limited constructed person shut up in the formula of his own mechanism. This state of consciousness is so abnormal to our present mode of being that to the rational man who does not possess it it may seem impossible or even a state of alienation; but once possessed it vindicates itself even to the mental intelligence by its greater calm, freedom, light, power, effectivity of will, verifiable truth of ideation and feeling. For this condition begins already on the higher levels of liberated mind, and can therefore be partly sensed and understood by mind-intelligence, but it rises to perfect self-possession only when it leaves behind the mental levels, only in the supramental gnosis.

In this state of consciousness the infinite becomes to us the primal, the actual reality, the one thing immediately and sensibly true. It becomes impossible for us to think of or realise the finite apart from our fundamental sense of the infinite, in which alone the finite can live, can form itself, can have any reality or duration. So long as this finite mind and body are to our consciousness the first fact of our existence and the foundation of all our thinking, feeling and willing and so long as things finite are the normal reality from which we can rise occasionally, or even frequently, to an idea and sense of the infinite, we are still very far away from the gnosis. In the plane of the gnosis the infinite is at once our normal consciousness of being, its first fact, our sensible substance. It is very concretely to us there the foundation from which everything finite forms itself and its boundless incalculable forces are the origination of all our thought, will and delight. But this infinite is not only an infinite of pervasion or of extension in which everything forms and happens. Behind that immeasurable extension the gnostic consciousness is always aware of a spaceless inner infinite. It is through this double infinite that we shall arrive at the essential being of Sachchidananda, the highest self of our own being and the totality of our cosmic existence. There is opened to us an illimitable existence which we feel as if it were an infinity above us to which we attempt to rise and an infinity around us into which we strive to dissolve our separate existence. Afterwards we widen into it and rise into it; we break out of the ego into its largeness and are that for ever. If this liberation is achieved, its power can take, if so we will, increasing possession of our lower being also until even our lowest and perversest activities are refashioned into the truth of the Vijnana.

This is the basis, this sense of the infinite and possession by the infinite, and only when it is achieved, can we progress towards some normality of the supramental ideation, perception, sense, identity, awareness. For even this sense of the infinite is only a first foundation and much more has to be done before the consciousness can become dynamically gnostic. The supramental knowledge is the play of a supreme light; there are many other lights, other levels of knowledge higher than human mind which can open in us and receive or reflect something of that effulgence even before we rise into the gnosis. But to command or wholly possess it we must first enter into and become the being of the supreme light, our consciousness must be transformed into that consciousness, its principle and power of self-awareness and all-awareness by identity must be the very stuff of our existence. For our means and ways of knowledge and action must necessarily be according to the nature of our consciousness and it is the consciousness that must radically change if we are to command and not only be occasionally visited by that higher power of knowledge. But it is not confined to a higher thought or the action of a sort of divine reason. It takes up all our present means of knowledge immensely extended, active and effective where they are now debarred, blind, infructuous, and turns them into a high and intense perceptive activity of the Vijnana. Thus it takes up our sense action and illumines it even in its ordinary field so that we get a true sense of things. But also it enables the mind-sense to have a direct perception of the inner as well as the outer phenomenon, to feel and receive or perceive, for instance, the thoughts, feelings, sensations, the nervous reactions of the object on which it is turned.[2] It uses the subtle senses as well as the physical and saves them from their errors. It gives us the knowledge, the experience of planes of existence other than the material to which our ordinary mentality is ignorantly attached and it enlarges the world for us. It transforms similarly the sensations and gives them their full intensity as well as their full holding-power; for in our normal mentality the full intensity is impossible because the power to hold and sustain vibrations beyond a certain point is denied to it, mind and body would both break under the shock or the prolonged strain. It takes up too the element of knowledge in our feelings and emotions,—for our feelings too contain a power of knowledge and a power of effectuation which we do not recognise and do not properly develop,—and delivers them at the same time from their limitations and from their errors and perversions. For in all things the gnosis is the Truth, the Right, the highest Law, *devānām adabdhāni vratāni*.

Knowledge and Force or Will—for all conscious force is will—are the twin sides of the action of consciousness. In our mentality they are divided. The idea comes first, the will comes stumbling after it or rebels against it or is used as its imperfect tool with imperfect results; or else the will starts up first with a blind or half-seeing idea in it and works out something in confusion of which we get the right understanding afterwards. There is no oneness, no full understanding between these powers in us; or else there is no perfect correspondence of initiation with effectuation. Nor is the individual will in harmony with the universal; it tries to reach beyond it or falls short of it or deviates from and strives against it. It knows not the times and seasons of the Truth, nor its degrees and measures. The Vijnana takes up the will and puts it first into harmony and then into oneness with the truth of the supramental knowledge. In this knowledge the idea in the individual is one with the idea in the universal, because both are brought back to the truth of the supreme Knowledge and the transcendent Will. The gnosis takes up not only our intelligent will, but our wishes, desires, even what we call the lower desires, the instincts, the impulses, the reachings out of sense and sensation and it transforms them. They cease to be wishes and desires, because they cease first to be personal and then cease to be that struggling after the ungrasped which we mean by craving and desire. No longer blind or half-blind reachings out of the instinctive or intelligent mentality, they are transformed into a various action of the Truth-will; and that will acts with an inherent knowledge of the right measures of its decreed action and therefore with an effectivity unknown to our mental willing. Therefore too in the action of the *vijñānamaya* will there is no place for sin; for all sin is an error of the will, a desire and act of the Ignorance.

When desire ceases entirely, grief and all inner suffering also cease. The Vijnana takes up not only our parts of knowledge and will, but our parts of affection and delight and changes them into action of the divine Ananda. For if knowledge and force are the twin sides or powers of the action of consciousness, delight, Ananda—which is something higher than what we call pleasure—is the very stuff of consciousness and the natural result of the interaction of knowledge and will, force and self-awareness. Both pleasure and pain, both joy and grief are deformations caused by the disturbance of harmony between our consciousness and the force it applies, between our knowledge and will, a breaking up of their oneness by a descent to a lower plane in which they are limited, divided in themselves, restrained from their full and proper action, at odds with other-force, other-consciousness, other-knowledge, other-will. The Vijnana sets this to rights by the power of its truth and a wholesale restoration to oneness and harmony, to the Right and the highest Law. It takes up all our emotions and turns them into various forms of love and delight, even our hatreds, repulsions, causes of suffering. It finds out or reveals the meaning they missed and by missing it became the perversions they are; it restores our whole nature to the eternal Good. It deals similarly with our perceptions and sensations and reveals all the delight that they seek, but in its truth, not in any perversion and wrong seeking and wrong reception; it teaches even our lower impulses to lay hold on the Divine and Infinite in the appearances after which they run. All this is done not in the values of the lower being, but by a lifting up of the mental, vital, material into the inalienable purity, the natural intensity, the continual ecstasy, one yet manifold, of the divine Ananda.

Thus the being of Vijnana is in all its activities a play of perfected knowledge-power, will-power, delight-power, raised to a higher than the mental, vital and bodily level. All-pervasive, universalised, freed from egoistic personality and individuality, it is the play of a higher Self, a higher consciousness and therefore a higher force and higher delight of being. All that acts in the Vijnana in the purity, in the right, in the truth of the superior or divine Prakriti. Its powers may often seem to be what are called in ordinary Yogic parlance siddhis, by the Europeans occult powers, shunned and dreaded by devotees and by many Yogins as snares, stumbling-blocks, diversions from the true seeking after the Divine. But they have that character and are dangerous here because they are sought in the lower being, abnormally, by the ego for an egoistic satisfaction. In the Vijnana they are neither occult nor siddhis, but the open, unforced and normal play of its nature. The Vijnana is the Truth-power and Truth-action of the divine Being in its divine identities, and, when this acts through the individual lifted to the gnostic plane, it fulfils itself unperverted, without fault or egoistic reaction, without diversion from the possession of the Divine. There the individual is no longer the ego, but the free Jiva domiciled in the higher divine nature of which he is a portion, *parā prakṛtir jīvabhūtā*, the nature of the supreme and universal Self seen indeed in the play of multiple individuality out without the veil of ignorance, with self-knowledge, in its multiple oneness, in the truth of its divine Shakti.

In the Vijnana the right relation and action of Purusha and Prakriti are found, because there they become unified and the Divine is no longer veiled in Maya. All is his action. The Jiva no longer says "I think, I act, I desire, I feel"; he does not even say like the sadhaka striving after unity but before he has reached it, "As appointed by Thee seated in my heart, I act." For the heart, the centre of the mental consciousness is no longer the centre of origination but only a blissful channel. He is rather aware of the Divine seated above, lord of all, *adhiṣṭhita*, as well as acting within him. And seated himself in that higher being, *parārdhe, paramasyāṁ parāvati*, he can say truly and boldly, "God himself by his Prakriti knows, acts, loves, takes delight through my individuality and its figures and fulfils there in its higher and divine measures the multiple *līlā* which the Infinite for ever plays in the universality which is himself for ever."

---

1. Many, if not all, of these conditions of the gnostic change can and indeed have to be attained long before we reach the gnosis,—but imperfectly at first as if by a reflection, —in higher mind itself, and more completely in what we may call an over-mind consciousness between mentality and gnosis.
2. This power, says Patanjali, comes by "*saṁyama*" on an object. That is for the mentality, in the gnosis there is no need of *saṁyama*. For this kind of perception is the natural action of the Vijnana.

# GNOSIS AND ANANDA

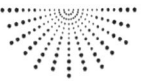

THE ASCENT to the gnosis, the possession of something of the gnostic consciousness must elevate the soul of man and sublimate his life in the world into a glory of light and power and bliss and infinity that can seem in comparison with the lame action and limited realisations of our present mental and physical existence the very status and dynamis of a perfection final and absolute. And it is a true perfection, such as nothing before it has yet been in the ascension of the spirit. For even the highest spiritual realisation on the plane of mentality has in it something top-heavy, one-sided and exclusive; even the widest mental spirituality is not wide enough and it is marred too by its imperfect power of self-expression in life. And yet in comparison with what is beyond it, this too, this first gnostic splendour is only a bright passage to a more perfect perfection. It is the secure and shining step from which we can happily mount still upwards into the absolute infinities which are the origin and the goal of the incarnating spirit. In this farther ascension the gnosis does not disappear, but reaches rather its own supreme Light out of which it has descended to mediate between mind and the supreme Infinite.

The Upanishad tells us that after the knowledge-self above the mental is possessed and all the lower selves have been drawn up into it, there is another and last step of all still left to us—though one might ask, is it eternally the last or only the last practically conceivable or at all necessary for us now?—to take up our gnostic existence into the Bliss-Self and there complete the spiritual self-discovery of the divine Infinite. Ananda, a supreme Bliss eternal, far other and higher in its character than the highest human joy or pleasure, is the essential and original nature of the spirit. In Ananda our spirit will find its true self, in Ananda its essential consciousness, in Ananda the absolute power of its existence. The embodied soul's entry into this highest absolute, unlimited, unconditional bliss of the spirit is the infinite liberation and the infinite perfection. It is true that something of this bliss can be enjoyed by reflection, by a qualified descent even on the lower planes where the Purusha plays with his modified and qualified Nature. There can be the experience of a spiritual and boundless Ananda on the plane of matter, on the plane of life, on the plane of mind as well as on the gnostic truth-plane of knowledge and above it. And the Yogin who enters into these lesser realisations, may find them so complete and compelling that he will imagine there is nothing greater, nothing beyond it. For each of the divine principles contains in itself the whole potentiality of all the other six notes of our being; each plane of Nature can have its own perfection of these notes under its own conditions. But the integral perfection can come only by a mounting ascent of the lowest into the highest and an incessant descent of the highest into the lowest till all becomes one at once solid block and plastic sea-stuff of the Truth infinite and eternal.

The very physical consciousness in man, the *annamaya puruṣa*, can without this supreme ascent and integral descent yet reflect and enter into the self of Sachchidananda. It can do it either by a reflection of the Soul in physical Nature, its bliss, power and infinity secret but still present here, or by losing its separate sense of substance and existence in the Self within or without it. The result is a glorified sleep of the physical mind in which the physical being forgets itself in a kind of conscious Nirvana or else moves about like a thing inert in the hands of Nature, *jaḍavat*, like a leaf in the wind, or otherwise a state of pure happy and free irresponsibility of action, *bālavat*, a divine childhood. But this comes without the higher glories of knowledge and delight which belong to the same status upon a more exalted level. It is an inert realisation of Sachchidananda in which there is neither any mastery of the Prakriti by the Purusha nor any sublimation of Nature into her own supreme power, the infinite glories of the Para Shakti. Yet these two, this mastery and this sublimation, are the two gates of perfection, the splendid doors into the supreme Eternal.

The life soul and life consciousness in man, *prāṇamaya puruṣa*, can in the same way directly reflect and enter into the self of Sachchidananda by a large and splendid and blissful reflection of the Soul in universal Life or by losing its separate sense of life and existence in the vast Self within or without it. The result is either a profound state of sheer self-oblivion or else an action driven irresponsibly by the life nature, an exalted enthusiasm of self-abandonment to the great world-energy in its vitalistic dance. The outer being lives in a God-possessed frenzy careless of itself and the world, *unmattavat*, or with an entire disregard whether of the conventions and proprieties of fitting human action or of the harmony and rhythms of a greater Truth. It acts as the unbound vital being, *piśācavat*, the divine maniac or else the divine demoniac. Here too there is no mastery or supreme sublimation of nature. There is only a joyful static possession by the Self within us and an unregulated dynamic possession by the physical and the vital Nature without us.

The mind soul and mind consciousness in man, *manomaya puruṣa*, can in the same direct way reflect and enter into Sachchidananda by a reflection of the Soul as it mirrors itself in the nature of pure universal mind luminous, unwalled, happy, plastic, illimitable, or by absorption in the vast free unconditioned uncentred Self within it and without it. The result is either the immobile cessation of all mind and action or a desire-free unbound action watched by the unparticipating inner Witness. The mental being becomes the eremite soul alone in the world and careless of all human ties or the saint soul that lives in a rapturous God-nearness or felicitous identity and in joyful relations of pure love and ecstasy towards all creatures. The mental being may even realise the Self in all three planes together. Then he is all these things alternately, successively or at once. Or he may transform the lower forms into manifestations of the higher state; he may draw upward the childlikeness or the inert irresponsibility of the free physical mind or the free vital mind's divine madness and carelessness of all rules, proprieties, harmonies and colour or disguise with them the ecstasy of the saint or the solitary liberty of the wandering eremite. Here again there is no mastery, no sublimation of the Nature by the soul in the world, but a double possession, by the freedom and delight of the mental-spiritual infinite within and without by the happy, natural and unregulated play of the mind-Nature. But since the mental being is capable of receiving the gnosis in a way in which the life soul and physical soul cannot receive it, since he can accept it with knowledge though only the limited knowledge of a mental response, he may to a certain extent govern by its light his outer action or, if not that, at least bathe and purify in it his will and his thinkings. But Mind can arrive only at a compromise between the infinite within and the finite nature without; it cannot pour the infinity of the inner being's knowledge and power and bliss with any sense of fullness into its external action which remains always inadequate. Still it is content and free because it is the Lord within who takes up the responsibility of the action adequate or inadequate, assumes its guidance and fixes its consequence.

But the gnostic soul, the *vijñānamaya puruṣa*, is the first to participate not only in the freedom, but in the power and sovereignty of the Eternal. For it receives the fullness, it has the sense of plenitude of the Godhead in its action; it shares the free, splendid and royal march of the Infinite, is a vessel of the original knowledge, the immaculate power, the inviolable bliss, transmutes all life into the eternal Light and the eternal Fire and the eternal Wine of the nectar. It possesses the infinite of the Self and it possesses the infinite of Nature. It does not so much lose as find its nature self in the self of the Infinite. On the other planes to which the mental being has easier access, man finds God in himself and himself in God; he becomes divine in essence rather than in person or nature. In the gnosis, even the mentalised gnosis, the Divine Eternal possesses, changes and stamps the human symbol, envelops and partly finds himself in the person and nature. The mental being at most receives or reflects that which is true, divine and eternal; the gnostic soul reaches a true identity, possesses the spirit and power of the truth-Nature. In the gnosis the dualism of Purusha and Prakriti, Soul and Nature, two separate powers complementary to each other, the great truth of the Sankhyas founded on the practical truth of our present natural existence, disappears in their biune entity, the dynamic mystery of the occult Supreme. The Truth-being is the Hara-Gauri[1] of the Indian iconological symbol; it is the double Power masculine-feminine born from and supported by the supreme Shakti of the Supreme.

Therefore the truth-soul does not arrive at self-oblivion in the Infinite; it comes to an eternal self-possession in the Infinite. Its action is not irregular; it is a perfect control in an infinite freedom. In the lower planes the soul is naturally subject to Nature and the regulating principle is found in the lower nature; all regulation there depends on the acceptance of a strict subjection to the law of the finite. If the soul on these planes withdraws from that law into the liberty of the infinite, it loses its natural centre and becomes centreless in a cosmic infinitude; it forfeits the living harmonic principle by which its external being was till then regulated and it finds no other. The personal nature or what is left of it merely continues mechanically for a while its past movements, or it dances in the gusts and falls of the universal energy that acts on the individual system rather than in that system, or it strays in the wild steps of an irresponsible ecstasy, or it remains inert and abandoned by the breath of the Spirit that was within it. If on the other hand the soul moves in its impulse of freedom towards the discovery of another and divine centre of control through which the Infinite can consciously govern its own action in the individual, it is moving towards the gnosis where that centre pre-exists, the centre of an eternal harmony and order. It is when he ascends above mind and life to the gnosis that the Purusha becomes the master of his own nature because subject only to supreme Nature. For there force or will is the exact counterpart, the perfect dynamis of the divine knowledge. And that knowledge is not merely the eye of the Witness, it is the immanent and compelling gaze of the Ishwara. Its luminous governing power, a power not to be hedged in or denied, imposes its self-expressive force on all the action and makes true and radiant and authentic and inevitable every movement and impulse.

The gnosis does not reject the realisations of the lower planes; for it is not an annihilation or extinction, not a Nirvana but a sublime fulfilment of our manifested Nature. It possesses the first realisations under its own conditions after it has transformed them and made them elements of a divine order. The gnostic soul is the child, but the king-child;[2] here is the royal and eternal childhood whose toys are the worlds and all universal Nature is the miraculous garden of the play that tires never. The gnosis takes up the condition of divine inertia; but this is no longer the inertia of the subject soul driven by Nature like a fallen leaf in the breath of the Lord. It is the happy passivity bearing an unimaginable intensity of action and Ananda of the Nature-Soul at once driven by the bliss of the mastering Purusha and aware of herself as the supreme Shakti above and around him and mastering and carrying him blissfully on her bosom for ever. This biune being of Purusha-Prakriti is as if a flaming Sun and body of divine Light self-carried in its orbit by its own inner consciousness and power at one with the universal, at one with a supreme Transcendence. Its madness is a wise madness of Ananda, the incalculable ecstasy of a supreme consciousness and power vibrating with an infinite sense of freedom and intensity in its divine life-movements. Its action is supra-rational and therefore to the rational mind which has not the key it seems a colossal madness. And yet this that seems madness is a wisdom in action that only baffles the mind by the liberty and richness of its contents and the infinite complexity in fundamental simplicity of its motions, it is the very method of the Lord of the worlds, a thing no intellectual interpretation can fathom,—a dance this also, a whirl of mighty energies, but the Master of the dance holds the hands of His energies and keeps them to the rhythmic order, the self-traced harmonic circles of his Rasa-lila. The gnostic soul is not bound any more than the divine demoniac by the petty conventions and proprieties of the normal human life or the narrow rules through which it makes some shift to accommodate itself with the perplexing dualities of the lower nature and tries to guide its steps among the seeming contradictions of the world, to avoid its numberless stumbling-blocks and to foot with gingerly care around its dangers and pitfalls. The gnostic supramental life is abnormal to us because it is free to all the hardihoods and audacious delights of a soul dealing fearlessly and even violently with Nature, but yet is it the very normality of the infinite and all governed by the law of the Truth in its exact unerring process. It obeys the law of a self-possessed Knowledge, Love, Delight in an innumerable Oneness. It seems abnormal only because its rhythm is not measurable by the faltering beats of the mind, but yet it steps in a wonderful and transcendent measure.

And what then is the necessity of a still higher step and what difference is there between the soul in gnosis and the soul in the Bliss? There is no essential difference, but yet a difference, because there is a transfer to another consciousness and a certain reversal in position,—for at each step of the ascent from Matter to the highest Existence there is a reversal of consciousness. The soul no longer looks up to something beyond it, but is in it and from it looks down on all that it was before. On all planes indeed the Ananda can be discovered, because everywhere it exists and is the same. Even there is a repetition of the Ananda plane in each lower world of consciousness. But in the lower planes not only is it reached by a sort of dissolution into it of the pure mind or the life-sense or the physical awareness, but it is, as it were, itself diluted by the dissolved form of mind, life or matter, held in the dilution and turned into a poor thinness wonderful to the lower consciousness but not comparable to its true intensities. The gnosis has on the contrary a dense light of essential consciousness[3] in which the intense fullness of the Ananda can be. And when the form of gnosis is dissolved into the Ananda, it is not annulled altogether, but undergoes a natural change by which the soul is carried up into its last and absolute freedom; for it casts itself into the absolute existence of the spirit and is enlarged into its own entirely self-existent bliss infinitudes. The gnosis has the infinite and absolute as the conscious source, accompaniment, condition, standard, field and atmosphere of all its activities, it possesses it as its base, fount, constituent material, indwelling and inspiring Presence; but in its action it seems to stand out from it as its operation, as the rhythmical working of its activities, as a divine Maya[4] or Wisdom-Formation of the Eternal. Gnosis is the divine Knowledge-Will of the divine Consciousness-Force; it is harmonic consciousness and action of Prakriti-Purusha full of the delight of the divine existence. In the Ananda the knowledge goes back from these willed harmonies into pure self-consciousness, the will dissolves into pure transcendent force and both are taken up into the pure delight of the Infinite. The basis of the gnostic existence is the self-stuff and self-form of the Ananda.

This in the ascension takes place because there is here completed the transition to the absolute unity of which the gnosis is the decisive step, but not the final resting-place. In the gnosis the soul is aware of its infinity and lives in it, yet it lives also in a working centre for the individual play of the Infinite. It realises its identity with all existences, but it keeps a distinction without difference by which it can have also the contact with them in a certain diverseness. This is that distinction for the joy of contact which in the mind becomes not only difference, but in its self-experience division from our other selves, in its spiritual being a sense of loss of self one with us in others and a reaching after the felicity it has forfeited, in life a compromise between egoistic self-absorption and a blind seeking out for the lost oneness. In its infinite consciousness, the gnostic soul creates a sort of voluntary limitation for its own wisdom-purposes; it has even its particular luminous aura of being in which it moves, although beyond that it enters into all things and identifies itself with all being and all existences. In the Ananda all is reversed, the centre disappears. In the bliss nature there is no centre, nor any voluntary or imposed circumference, but all is, all are one equal being, one identical spirit. The bliss soul finds and feels itself everywhere; it has no mansion, is *aniketa*, or has the all for its mansion, or, if it likes, it has all things for its many mansions open to each other for ever. All other selves are entirely its own selves, in action as well as in essence. The joy of contact in diverse oneness becomes altogether the joy of absolute identity in innumerable oneness. Existence is no longer formulated in the terms of the Knowledge, because the known and knowledge and the knower are wholly one self here and, since all possesses all in an intimate identity beyond the closest closeness, there is no need of what we call knowledge. All the consciousness is of the bliss of the Infinite, all power is power of the bliss of the Infinite, all forms and activities are forms and activities of the bliss of the Infinite. In this absolute truth of its being the eternal soul of Ananda lives, here deformed by contrary phenomena, there brought back and transfigured into their reality.

The soul lives: it is not abolished, it is not lost in a featureless Indefinite. For on every plane of our existence the same principle holds; the soul may fall asleep in a trance of self-absorption, dwell in an ineffable intensity of God-possession, live in the highest glory of its own plane,— the Anandaloka, Brahmaloka, Vaikuntha, Goloka of various Indian systems,—even turn upon the lower worlds to fill them with its own light and power and beatitude. In the eternal worlds and more and more in all worlds above Mind these states exist in each other. For they are not separate; they are coexistent, even coincident powers of the consciousness of the Absolute. The Divine on the Ananda plane is not incapable of a world-play or self-debarred from any expression of its glories. On the contrary, as the Upanishad insists, the Ananda is the true creative principle. For all takes birth from this divine Bliss;[5] all is preexistent in it as an absolute truth of existence which the Vijnana brings out and subjects to voluntary limitation by the Idea and the law of the Idea. In the Ananda all law ceases and there is an absolute freedom without binding term or limit. It is superior to all principles and in one and the same motion the enjoyer of all principles; it is free from all gunas and the enjoyer of its own infinite gunas; it is above all forms and the builder and enjoyer of all its self-forms and figures. This unimaginable completeness is what the spirit is, the spirit transcendent and universal, and to be one in bliss with the transcendent and universal spirit is for the soul too to be that and nothing less. Necessarily, since there is on this plane the absolute and the play of absolutes, it is ineffable by any of the conceptions of our mind or by signs of the phenomenal or ideal realities of which mind-conceptions are the figures in our intelligence. These realities are themselves indeed only relative symbols of those ineffable absolutes. The symbol, the expressive reality, may give an idea, a perception, sense, vision, contact even of the thing itself to us, but at last we get beyond it to the thing it symbolises, transcend idea, vision, contact, pierce through the ideal and pass to the real realities, the identical, the supreme, the timeless and eternal, the infinitely infinite.

Our first absorbing impulse when we become inwardly aware of something entirely beyond what we now are and know and are powerfully attracted to it, is to get away from the present actuality and dwell in that higher reality altogether. The extreme form of this attraction when we are drawn to the supreme Existence and the infinite Ananda is the condemnation of the lower and the finite as an illusion and an aspiration to Nirvana in the beyond,—the passion for dissolution, immersion, extinction in the Spirit. But the real dissolution, the true *nirvāṇa* is the release of all that is bindingly characteristic of the lower into the larger being of the Higher, the conscious possession of the living symbol by the living Real. We discover in the end that not only is that higher Reality the cause of all the rest, not only it embraces and exists in all the rest, but as more and more we possess it, all this rest is transformed in our soul-experience into a superior value and becomes the means of a richer expression of the Real, a more many-sided communion with the Infinite, a larger ascent to the Supreme. Finally, we get close to the absolute and its supreme values which are the absolutes of all things. We lose the passion for release, *mumukṣutva*, which till then actuated us, because we are now intimately near to that which is ever free, that which is neither attracted into attachment by what binds us now nor afraid of what to us seems to be bondage. It is only by the loss of the bound soul's exclusive passion for its freedom that there can come an absolute liberation of our nature. The Divine attracts the soul of man to him by various lures; all of them are born of its own relative and imperfect conceptions of bliss; all are its ways of seeking for the Ananda, but, if clung to till the end, miss the inexpressible truth of those surpassing felicities. First in order comes the lure of an earthly reward, a prize of material, intellectual, ethical or other joy in the terrestrial mind and body. A second remoter greater version of the same fruitful error is the hope of a heavenly bliss, far exceeding these earthly rewards; the conception of heaven rises in altitude and purity till it reaches the pure idea of the eternal presence of God or an unending union with the Eternal. And last we get the subtlest of all lures, an escape from these worldly or heavenly joys and from all pains and sorrows, effort and trouble and from all phenomenal things, a Nirvana, a self-dissolution in the Absolute, an Ananda of cessation and ineffable peace. In the end all these toys of the mind have to be transcended. The fear of birth and the desire of escape from birth must entirely fall away from us. For, to repeat the ancient language, the soul that has realised oneness has no sorrow or shrinking; the spirit that has entered into the bliss of the Spirit has nought to fear from anyone or anything whatsoever. Fear, desire and sorrow are diseases of the mind; born of its sense of division and limitation, they cease with the falsehood that begot them. The Ananda is free from these maladies; it is not the monopoly of the ascetic, it is not born from the disgust of existence.

The bliss soul is not bound to birth or to non-birth; it is not driven by desire of the Knowledge or harassed by fear of the Ignorance. The supreme bliss Soul has already the Knowledge and transcends all need of knowledge. Not limited in consciousness by the form and the act, it can play with the manifestation without being imbued with the Ignorance. Already it is taking its part above in the mystery of an eternal manifestation and here, when the time comes, it will descend into birth without being the slave of Ignorance chained to the revolutions of the wheel of Nature. For it knows that the purpose and law of the birth-series is for the soul in the body to rise from plane to plane and substitute always the rule of the higher for the rule of the lower play even down to the material field. The bliss-soul neither disdains to help that ascent from above nor fears to descend down the stairs of God into the material birth and there contribute the power of its own bliss nature to the upward pull of the divine forces. The time for that marvellous hour of the evolving Time-Spirit is not yet come. Man, generally, cannot yet ascend to the bliss nature; he has first to secure himself on the higher mental altitudes, to ascend from them to the gnosis. Still less can he bring down all the Bliss-Power into this terrestrial Nature; he must first cease to be mental man and become superhuman. All he can do now is to receive something of its power into his soul in greater or less degree, by a diminishing transmission through an inferior consciousness; but even that gives him the sense of an ecstasy and an unsurpassable beatitude.

And what will be the bliss nature when it manifests in a new supramental race? The fully evolved soul will be one with all beings in the status and dynamic effects of experience of a bliss-consciousness intense and illimitable. And since love is the effective power and soul-symbol of bliss-oneness he will approach and enter into this oneness by the gate of universal love, a sublimation of human love at first, a divine love afterwards, at its summits a thing of beauty, sweetness and splendour now to us inconceivable. He will be one in bliss-consciousness with all the world-play and its powers and happenings and there will be banished for ever the sorrow and fear, the hunger and pain of our poor and darkened mental and vital and physical existence. He will get that power of the bliss-freedom in which all the conflicting principles of our being shall be unified in their absolute values. All evil shall perforce change itself into good; the universal beauty of the All-beautiful will take possession of its fallen kingdoms; every darkness will be converted into a pregnant glory of light and the discords which the mind creates between Truth and Good and Beauty, Power and Love and Knowledge will disappear on the eternal summit, in the infinite extensions where they are always one.

The Purusha in mind, life and body is divided from Nature and in conflict with her. He labours to control and coerce what he can embody of her by his masculine force and is yet subject to her afflicting dualities and in fact her plaything from top to bottom, beginning to end. In the gnosis he is biune with her, finds as master of his own nature their reconciliation and harmony by their essential oneness even while he accepts an infinite blissful subjection, the condition of his mastery and his liberties, to the Supreme in his sovereign divine Nature. In the tops of the gnosis and in the Ananda he is one with the Prakriti and no longer solely biune with her. There is no longer the baffling play of Nature with the soul in the Ignorance; all is the conscious play of the soul with itself and all its selves and the Supreme and the divine Shakti in its own and the infinite bliss nature. This is the supreme mystery, the highest secret, simple to its own experience, however difficult and complex to our mental conceptions and the effort of our limited intelligence to understand what is beyond it. In the free infinity of the self-delight of Sachchidananda there is a play of the divine Child, a *rāsa līlā* of the infinite Lover and its mystic soul-symbols repeat themselves in characters of beauty and movements and harmonies of delight in a timeless forever.

---

1. The biune body of the Lord and his Spouse, Ishwara and Shakti, the right half male, the left half female.
2. So Heraclitus, "The kingdom is of the child."
3. *cidghana*.
4. Not in the sense of illusion, but in the original Vedic significance of the word Maya. All in the gnostic existence is real, spiritually concrete, eternally verifiable.
5. Therefore the world of the Ananda is called the Janaloka, in the double sense of birth and delight.

# THE HIGHER AND THE LOWER
# KNOWLEDGE

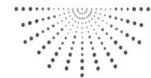

WE HAVE now completed our view of the path of Knowledge and seen to what it leads. First, the end of Yoga of Knowledge is God-possession, it is to possess God and be possessed by him through consciousness, through identification, through reflection of the divine Reality. But not merely in some abstraction away from our present existence, but here also; therefore to possess the Divine in himself, the Divine in the world, the Divine within, the Divine in all things and all beings. It is to possess oneness with God and through that to possess also oneness with the universal, with the cosmos and all existences; therefore to possess the infinite diversity also in the oneness, but on the basis of oneness and not on the basis of division. It is to possess God in his personality and his impersonality; in his purity free from qualities and in his infinite qualities; in time and beyond time; in his action and in his silence; in the finite and in the infinite. It is to possess him not only in pure self, but in all self; not only in self, but in Nature; not only in spirit, but in supermind, mind, life and body; to possess him with the spirit, with the mind, with the vital and the physical consciousness; and it is again for all these to be possessed by him, so that our whole being is one with him, full of him, governed and driven by him. It is, since God is oneness, for our physical consciousness to be one with the soul and the nature of the material universe; for our life, to be one with all life; for our mind, to be one with the universal mind; for our spirit, to be identified with the universal spirit. It is to merge in him in the absolute and find him in all relations.

Secondly, it is to put on the divine being and the divine nature. And since God is Sachchidananda, it is to raise our being into the divine being, our consciousness into the divine consciousness, our energy into the divine energy, our delight of existence into the divine delight of being. And it is not only to lift ourselves into this higher consciousness, but to widen into it in all our being, because it is to be found on all the planes of our existence and in all our members, so that our mental, vital, physical existence shall become full of the divine nature. Our intelligent mentality is to become a play of the divine knowledge-will, our mental soul-life a play of the divine love and delight, our vitality a play of the divine life, our physical being a mould of the divine substance. This God-action in us is to be realised by an opening of ourselves to the divine gnosis and divine Ananda and, in its fullness, by an ascent into and a permanent dwelling in the gnosis and the Ananda. For though we live physically on the material plane and in normal outward-going life the mind and soul are preoccupied with material existence, this externality of our being is not a binding limitation. We can raise our internal consciousness from plane to plane of the relations of Purusha with Prakriti, and even become, instead of the mental being dominated by the physical soul and nature, the gnostic being or the bliss-self and assume the gnostic or the bliss nature. And by this raising of the inner life we can transform our whole outward-going existence; instead of a life dominated by matter we shall then have a life dominated by spirit with all its circumstances moulded and determined by the purity of being, the consciousness infinite even in the finite, the divine energy, the divine joy and bliss of the spirit.

This is the goal; we have seen also what are the essentials of the method. But here we have first to consider briefly one side of the question of method which we have hitherto left untouched. In the system of an integral Yoga the principle must be that all life is a part of the Yoga; but the knowledge which we have been describing seems to be not the knowledge of what is ordinarily understood as life, but of something behind life. There are two kinds of knowledge, that which seeks to understand the apparent phenomenon of existence externally, by an approach from outside, through the intellect,—this is the lower knowledge, the knowledge of the apparent world; secondly, the knowledge which seeks to know the truth of existence from within, in its source and reality, by spiritual realisation. Ordinarily, a sharp distinction is drawn between the two, and it is supposed that when we get to the higher knowledge, the God-knowledge, then the rest, the world-knowledge, becomes of no concern to us: but in reality they are two sides of one seeking. All knowledge is ultimately the knowledge of God, through himself, through Nature, through her works. Mankind has first to seek this knowledge through the external life; for until its mentality is sufficiently developed, spiritual knowledge is not really possible, and in proportion as it is developed, the possibilities of spiritual knowledge become richer and fuller.

Science, art, philosophy, ethics, psychology, the knowledge of man and his past, action itself are means by which we arrive at the knowledge of the workings of God through Nature and through life. At first it is the workings of life and forms of Nature which occupy us, but as we go deeper and deeper and get a completer view and experience, each of these lines brings us face to face with God. Science at its limits, even physical Science, is compelled to perceive in the end the infinite, the universal, the spirit, the divine intelligence and will in the material universe. Still more easily must this be the end with the psychic sciences which deal with the operations of higher and subtler planes and powers of our being and come into contact with the beings and the phenomena of the worlds behind which are unseen, not sensible by our physical organs, but ascertainable by the subtle mind and senses. Art leads to the same end; the aesthetic human being intensely preoccupied with Nature through aesthetic emotion must in the end arrive at spiritual emotion and perceive not only the infinite life, but the infinite presence within her; preoccupied with beauty in the life of man he must in the end come to see the divine, the universal, the spiritual in humanity. Philosophy dealing with the principles of things must come to perceive the Principle of all these principles and investigate its nature, attributes and essential workings. So ethics must eventually perceive that the law of good which it seeks is the law of God and depends on the being and nature of the Master of the law. Psychology leads from the study of mind and the soul in living beings to the perception of the one soul and one mind in all things and beings. The history and study of man like the history and study of Nature lead towards the perception of the eternal and universal Power and Being whose thought and will work out through the cosmic and human evolution. Action itself forces us into contact with the divine Power which works through, uses, overrules our actions. The intellect begins to perceive and understand, the emotions to feel and desire and revere, the will to turn itself to the service of the Divine without whom Nature and man cannot exist or move and by conscious knowledge of whom alone we can arrive at our highest possibilities.

It is here that Yoga steps in. It begins by using knowledge, emotion and action for the possession of the Divine. For Yoga is the conscious and perfect seeking of union with the Divine towards which all the rest was an ignorant and imperfect moving and seeking. At first, then, Yoga separates itself from the action and method of the lower knowledge. For while this lower knowledge approaches God indirectly from outside and never enters his secret dwelling-place, Yoga calls us within and approaches him directly; while that seeks him through the intellect and becomes conscious of him from behind a veil, Yoga seeks him through realisation, lifts the veil and gets the full vision; where that only feels the presence and the influence, Yoga enters into the presence and fills itself with the influence; where that is only aware of the workings and through them gets some glimpse of the Reality, Yoga identifies our inner being with the Reality and sees from that the workings. Therefore the methods of Yoga are different from the methods of the lower knowledge.

The method of Yoga in knowledge must always be a turning of the eye inward and, so far as it looks upon outer things, a penetrating of the surface appearances to get at the one eternal reality within them. The lower knowledge is preoccupied with the appearances and workings; it is the first necessity of the higher to get away from them to the Reality of which they are the appearances and the Being and Power of conscious existence of which they are the workings. It does this by three movements each necessary to each other, by each of which the others become complete,—purification, concentration, identification. The object of purification is to make the whole mental being a clear mirror in which the divine reality can be reflected, a clear vessel and an unobstructing channel into which the divine presence and through which the divine influence can be poured, a subtilised stuff which the divine nature can take possession of, new-shape and use to divine issues. For the mental being at present reflects only the confusions created by the mental and physical view of the world, is a channel only for the disorders of the ignorant lower nature and full of obstructions and impurities which prevent the higher from acting; therefore the whole shape of our being is deformed and imperfect, indocile to the highest influences and turned in its action to ignorant and inferior utilities. It reflects even the world falsely; it is incapable of reflecting the Divine.

Concentration is necessary, first, to turn the whole will and mind from the discursive divagation natural to them, following a dispersed movement of the thoughts, running after many-branching desires, led away in the track of the senses and the outward mental response to phenomena: we have to fix the will and the thought on the eternal and real behind all, and this demands an immense effort, a one-pointed concentration. Secondly, it is necessary in order to break down the veil which is erected by our ordinary mentality between ourselves and the truth; for outer knowledge can be picked up by the way, by ordinary attention and reception, but the inner, hidden and higher truth can only be seized by an absolute concentration of the mind on its object, an absolute concentration of the will to attain it and, once attained, to hold it habitually and securely unite oneself with it. For identification is the condition of complete knowledge and possession; it is the intense result of a habitual purified reflecting of the reality and an entire concentration on it; and it is necessary in order to break down entirely that division and separation of ourselves from the divine being and the eternal reality which is the normal condition of our unregenerated ignorant mentality.

None of these things can be done by the methods of the lower knowledge. It is true that here also they have a preparing action, but up to a certain point and to a certain degree of intensity only, and it is where their action ceases that the action of Yoga takes up our growth into the Divine and finds the means to complete it. All pursuit of knowledge, if not vitiated by a too earthward tendency, tends to refine, to subtilise, to purify the being. In proportion as we become more mental, we attain to a subtler action of our whole nature which becomes more apt to reflect and receive higher thoughts, a purer will, a less physical truth, more inward influences. The power of ethical knowledge and the ethical habit of thought and will to purify is obvious. Philosophy not only purifies the reason and predisposes it to the contact of the universal and the infinite, but tends to stabilise the nature and create the tranquillity of the sage; and tranquillity is a sign of increasing self-mastery and purity. The preoccupation with universal beauty even in its aesthetic forms has an intense power for refining and subtilising the nature, and at its highest it is a great force for purification. Even the scientific habit of mind and the disinterested preoccupation with cosmic law and truth not only refine the reasoning and observing faculty, but have, when not counteracted by other tendencies, a steadying, elevating and purifying influence on the mind and moral nature which has not been sufficiently noticed.

The concentration of the mind and the training of the will towards the reception of the truth and living in the truth is also an evident result, a perpetual necessity of these pursuits; and at the end or in their highest intensities they may and do lead first to an intellectual, then to a reflective perception of the divine Reality which may culminate in a sort of preliminary identification with it. But all this cannot go beyond a certain point. The systematic purification of the whole being for an integral reflection and taking in of the divine reality can only be done by the special methods of Yoga. Its absolute concentration has to take the place of the dispersed concentrations of the lower knowledge; the vague and ineffective identification which is all the lower knowledge can bring, has to be replaced by the complete, intimate, imperative and living union which Yoga brings.

Nevertheless, Yoga does not either in its path or in its attainment exclude and throw away the forms of the lower knowledge, except when it takes the shape of an extreme asceticism or a mysticism altogether intolerant of this other divine mystery of the world-existence. It separates itself from them by the intensity, largeness and height of its objective and the specialisation of its methods to suit its aim; but it not only starts from them, but for a certain part of the way carries them with it and uses them as auxiliaries. Thus it is evident how largely ethical thought and practice,—not so much external as internal conduct,—enter into the preparatory method of Yoga, into its aim at purity. Again the whole method of Yoga is psychological; it might almost be termed the consummate practice of a perfect psychological knowledge. The data of philosophy are the supports from which it begins in the realisation of God through the principles of his being; only it carries the intelligent understanding which is all philosophy gives, into an intensity which carries it beyond thought into vision and beyond understanding into realisation and possession; what philosophy leaves abstract and remote, it brings into a living nearness and spiritual concreteness. The aesthetic and emotional mind and aesthetic forms are used by Yoga as a support for concentration even in the Yoga of knowledge and are, sublimated, the whole means of the Yoga of love and delight, as life and action, sublimated, are the whole means of the Yoga of works. Contemplation of God in Nature, contemplation and service of God in man and in the life of man and of the world in its past, present and future, are equally elements of which the Yoga of knowledge can make use to complete the realisation of God in all things. Only, all is directed to the one aim, directed towards God, filled with the idea of the divine, infinite, universal existence so that the outward-going, sensuous, pragmatical preoccupation of the lower knowledge with phenomena and forms is replaced by the one divine preoccupation. After attainment the same character remains. The Yogin continues to know and see God in the finite and be a channel of God-consciousness and God-action in the world; therefore the knowledge of the world and the enlarging and uplifting of all that appertains to life comes within his scope. Only, in all he sees God, sees the supreme reality, and his motive of work is to help mankind towards the knowledge of God and the possession of the supreme reality. He sees God through the data of science, God through the conclusions of philosophy, God through the forms of Beauty and the forms of Good, God in all the activities of life, God in the past of the world and its effects, in the present and its tendencies, in the future and its great progression. Into any or all of these he can bring his illumined vision and his liberated power of the spirit. The lower knowledge has been the step from which he has risen to the higher; the higher illumines for him the lower and makes it part of itself, even if only its lower fringe and most external radiation.

# SAMADHI

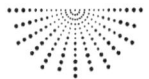

INTIMATELY connected with the aim of the Yoga of Knowledge which must always be the growth, the ascent or the withdrawal into a higher or a divine consciousness not now normal to us, is the importance attached to the phenomenon of Yogic trance, to Samadhi. It is supposed that there are states of being which can only be gained in trance; that especially is to be desired in which all action of awareness is abolished and there is no consciousness at all except the pure supramental immersion in immobile, timeless and infinite being. By passing away in this trance the soul departs into the silence of the highest Nirvana without possibility of return into any illusory or inferior state of existence. Samadhi is not so all-important in the Yoga of devotion, but it still has its place there as the swoon of being into which the ecstasy of divine love casts the soul. To enter into it is the supreme step of the ladder of Yogic practice in Rajayoga and Hathayoga. What then is the nature of Samadhi or the utility of its trance in an integral Yoga? It is evident that where our objective includes the possession of the Divine in life, a state of cessation of life cannot be the last consummating step or the highest desirable condition: Yogic trance cannot be an aim, as in so many Yogic systems, but only a means, and a means not of escape from the waking existence, but to enlarge and raise the whole seeing, living and active consciousness.

The importance of Samadhi rests upon the truth which modern knowledge is rediscovering, but which has never been lost in Indian psychology, that only a small part whether of world-being or of our own being comes into our ken or into our action. The rest is hidden behind in subliminal reaches of being which descend into the profoundest depths of the subconscient and rise to highest peaks of superconscience, or which surround the little field of our waking self with a wide circumconscient existence of which our mind and sense catch only a few indications. The old Indian psychology expressed this fact by dividing consciousness into three provinces, waking state, dream-state, sleep-state, *jāgrat, svapna, suṣupti*; and it supposed in the human being a waking self, a dream-self, a sleep-self, with the supreme or absolute self of being, the fourth or Turiya, beyond, of which all these are derivations for the enjoyment of relative experience in the world.

If we examine the phraseology of the old books, we shall find that the waking state is the consciousness of the material universe which we normally possess in this embodied existence dominated by the physical mind. The dream-state is a consciousness corresponding to the subtler life-plane and mind-plane behind, which to us, even when we get intimations of them, have not the same concrete reality as the things of the physical existence. The sleep-state is a consciousness corresponding to the supramental plane proper to the gnosis, which is beyond our experience because our causal body or envelope of gnosis is not developed in us, its faculties not active, and therefore we are in relation to that plane in a condition of dreamless sleep. The Turiya beyond is the consciousness of our pure self-existence or our absolute being with which we have no direct relations at all, whatever mental reflections we may receive in our dream or our waking or even, irrecoverably, in our sleep consciousness. This fourfold scale corresponds to the degrees of the ladder of being by which we climb back towards the absolute Divine. Normally therefore we cannot get back from the physical mind to the higher planes or degrees of consciousness without receding from the waking state, without going in and away from it and losing touch with the material world. Hence to those who desire to have the experience of these higher degrees, trance becomes a desirable thing, a means of escape from the limitations of the physical mind and nature.

Samadhi or Yogic trance retires to increasing depths according as it draws farther and farther away from the normal or waking state and enters into degrees of consciousness less and less communicable to the waking mind, less and less ready to receive a summons from the waking world. Beyond a certain point the trance becomes complete and it is then almost or quite impossible to awaken or call back the soul that has receded into them; it can only come back by its own will or at most by a violent shock of physical appeal dangerous to the system owing to the abrupt upheaval of return. There are said to be supreme states of trance in which the soul persisting for too long a time cannot return; for it loses its hold on the cord which binds it to the consciousness of life, and the body is left, maintained indeed in its set position, not dead by dissolution, but incapable of recovering the ensouled life which had inhabited it. Finally, the Yogin acquires at a certain stage of development the power of abandoning his body definitively without the ordinary phenomena of death, by an act of will,[1] or by a process of withdrawing the pranic life-force through the gate of the upward life-current (*udāna*), opening for it a way through the mystic *brahmarandhra* in the head. By departure from life in the state of Samadhi he attains directly to that higher status of being to which he aspires.

In the dream-state itself there are an infinite series of depths; from the lighter recall is easy and the world of the physical senses is at the doors, though for the moment shut out; in the deeper it becomes remote and less able to break in upon the inner absorption, the mind has entered into secure depths of trance. There is a complete difference between Samadhi and normal sleep, between the dream-state of Yoga and the physical state of dream. The latter belongs to the physical mind; in the former the mind proper and subtle is at work liberated from the immixture of the physical mentality. The dreams of the physical mind are an incoherent jumble made up partly of responses to vague touches from the physical world round which the lower mind-faculties disconnected from the will and reason, the *buddhi*, weave a web of wandering phantasy, partly of disordered associations from the brain-memory, partly of reflections from the soul travelling on the mental plane, reflections which are, ordinarily, received without intelligence or coordination, wildly distorted in the reception and mixed up confusedly with the other dream elements, with brain-memories and fantastic responses to any sensory touch from the physical world. In the Yogic dream-state, on the other hand, the mind is in clear possession of itself, though not of the physical world, works coherently and is able to use either its ordinary will and intelligence with a concentrated power or else the higher will and intelligence of the more exalted planes of mind. It withdraws from experience of the outer world, it puts its seals upon the physical senses and their doors of communication with material things; but everything that is proper to itself, thought, reasoning, reflection, vision, it can continue to execute with an increased purity and power of sovereign concentration free from the distractions and unsteadiness of the waking mind. It can use too its will and produce upon itself or upon its environment mental, moral and even physical effects which may continue and have their after consequences on the waking state subsequent to the cessation of the trance.

To arrive at full possession of the powers of the dream-state, it is necessary first to exclude the attack of the sights, sounds etc. of the outer world upon the physical organs. It is quite possible indeed to be aware in the dream-trance of the outer physical world through the subtle senses which belong to the subtle body; one may be aware of them just so far as one chooses and on a much wider scale than in the waking condition: for the subtle senses have a far more powerful range than the gross physical organs, a range which may be made practically unlimited. But this awareness of the physical world through the subtle senses is something quite different from our normal awareness of it through the physical organs; the latter is incompatible with the settled state of trance, for the pressure of the physical senses breaks the Samadhi and calls back the mind to live in their normal field where alone they have power. But the subtle senses have power both upon their own planes and upon the physical world, though this is to them more remote than their own world of being. In Yoga various devices are used to seal up the doors of the physical sense, some of them physical devices; but the one all-sufficient means is a force of concentration by which the mind is drawn inward to depths where the call of physical things can no longer easily attain to it. A second necessity is to get rid of the intervention of physical sleep. The ordinary habit of the mind when it goes in away from contact with physical things is to fall into the torpor of sleep or its dreams, and therefore when called in for the purposes of Samadhi, it gives or tends to give, at the first chance, by sheer force of habit, not the response demanded, but its usual response of physical slumber. This habit of the mind has to be got rid of; the mind has to learn to be awake in the dream-state, in possession of itself, not with the outgoing, but with an ingathered wakefulness in which, though immersed in itself, it exercises all its powers.

The experiences of the dream-state are infinitely various. For not only has it sovereign possession of the usual mental powers, reasoning, discrimination, will, imagination, and can use them in whatever way, on whatever subject, for whatever purpose it pleases, but it is able to establish connection with all the worlds to which it has natural access or to which it chooses to acquire access, from the physical to the higher mental worlds. This it does by various means open to the subtlety, flexibility and comprehensive movement of this internalised mind liberated from the narrow limitations of the physical outward-going senses. It is able first to take cognizance of all things whether in the material world or upon other planes by aid of perceptible images, not only images of things visible, but of sounds, touch, smell, taste, movement, action, of all that makes itself sensible to the mind and its organs. For the mind in Samadhi has access to the inner space called sometimes the *cidākāśa*, to depths of more and more subtle ether which are heavily curtained from the physical sense by the grosser ether of the material universe, and all things sensible, whether in the material world or any other, create reconstituting vibrations, sensible echoes, reproductions, recurrent images of themselves which that subtler ether receives and retains.

It is this which explains many of the phenomena of clairvoyance, clairaudience, etc.; for these phenomena are only the exceptional admission of the waking mentality into a limited sensitiveness to what might be called the image memory of the subtle ether, by which not only the signs of all things past and present, but even those of things future can be seized; for things future are already accomplished to knowledge and vision on higher planes of mind and their images can be reflected upon mind in the present. But these things which are exceptional to the waking mentality, difficult and to be perceived only by the possession of a special power or else after assiduous training, are natural to the dream-state of trance consciousness in which the subliminal mind is free. And that mind can also take cognizance of things on various planes not only by these sensible images, but by a species of thought perception or of thought reception and impression analogous to that phenomenon of consciousness which in modern psychical science has been given the name of telepathy. But the powers of the dream-state do not end here. It can by a sort of projection of ourselves, in a subtle form of the mental body, actually enter into other planes and worlds or into distant places and scenes of this world, move among them with a sort of bodily presence and bring back the direct experience of their scenes and truths and occurrences. It may even project actually the mental or vital body for the same purpose and travel in it, leaving the physical body in a profoundest trance without sign of life until its return.

The greatest value of the dream-state of Samadhi lies, however, not in these more outward things, but in its power to open up easily higher ranges and powers of thought, emotion, will by which the soul grows in height, range and self-mastery. Especially, withdrawing from the distraction of sensible things, it can, in a perfect power of concentrated self-seclusion, prepare itself by a free reasoning, thought, discrimination, or more intimately, more finally, by an ever deeper vision and identification, for access to the Divine, the supreme Self, the transcendent Truth, both in its principles and powers and manifestations and in its highest original Being. Or it can by an absorbed inner joy and emotion, as in a sealed and secluded chamber of the soul, prepare itself for the delight of union with the divine Beloved, the Master of all bliss, rapture and Ananda.

For the integral Yoga this method of Samadhi may seem to have the disadvantage that when it ceases, the thread is broken and the soul returns into the distraction and imperfection of the outward life, with only such an elevating effect upon that outer life as the general memory of these deeper experiences may produce. But this gulf, this break is not inevitable. In the first place, it is only in the untrained psychic being that the experiences of the trance are a blank to the waking mind; as it becomes the master of its Samadhi, it is able to pass without any gulf of oblivion from the inner to the outer waking. Secondly, when this has been once done, what is attained in the inner state, becomes easier to acquire by the waking consciousness and to turn into the normal experience, powers, mental status of the waking life. The subtle mind which is normally eclipsed by the insistence of the physical being, becomes powerful even in the waking state, until even there the enlarging man is able to live in his several subtle bodies as well as in his physical body, to be aware of them and in them, to use their senses, faculties, powers, to dwell in possession of supraphysical truth, consciousness and experience.

The sleep-state ascends to a higher power of being, beyond thought into pure consciousness, beyond emotion into pure bliss, beyond will into pure mastery; it is the gate of union with the supreme state of Sachchidananda out of which all the activities of the world are born. But here we must take care to avoid the pitfalls of symbolic language. The use of the words dream and sleep for these higher states is nothing but an image drawn from the experience of the normal physical mind with regard to planes in which it is not at home. It is not the truth that the Self in the third status called perfect sleep, *sus.upti*, is in a state of slumber. The sleep self is on the contrary described as Prajna, the Master of Wisdom and Knowledge, Self of the Gnosis, and as Ishwara, the Lord of being. To the physical mind a sleep, it is to our wider and subtler consciousness a greater waking. To the normal mind all that exceeds its normal experience but still comes into its scope, seems a dream; but at the point where it borders on things quite beyond its scope, it can no longer see truth even as in a dream, but passes into the blank incomprehension and non-reception of slumber. This border-line varies with the power of the individual consciousness, with the degree and height of its enlightenment and awakening. The line may be pushed up higher and higher until it may pass even beyond the mind. Normally indeed the human mind cannot be awake, even with the inner waking of trance, on the supramental levels; but this disability can be overcome. Awake on these levels the soul becomes master of the ranges of gnostic thought, gnostic will, gnostic delight, and if it can do this in Samadhi, it may carry its memory of experience and its power of experience over into the waking state. Even on the yet higher level open to us, that of the Ananda, the awakened soul may become similarly possessed of the Bliss-Self both in its concentration and in its cosmic comprehension. But still there may be ranges above from which it can bring back no memory except that which says, "somehow, indescribably, I was in bliss," the bliss of an unconditioned existence beyond all potentiality of expression by thought or description by image or feature. Even the sense of being may disappear in an experience in which the word existence loses its sense and the Buddhistic symbol of Nirvana seems alone and sovereignly justified. However high the power of awakening goes, there seems to be a beyond in which the image of sleep, of *suṣupti*, will still find its application.

Such is the principle of the Yogic trance, Samadhi,—into its complex phenomena we need not now enter. It is sufficient to note its double utility in the integral Yoga. It is true that up to a point difficult to define or delimit almost all that Samadhi can give, can be acquired without recourse to Samadhi. But still there are certain heights of spiritual and psychic experience of which the direct as opposed to a reflecting experience can only be acquired deeply and in its fullness by means of the Yogic trance. And even for that which can be otherwise acquired, it offers a ready means, a facility which becomes more helpful, if not indispensable, the higher and more difficult of access become the planes on which the heightened spiritual experience is sought. Once attained there, it has to be brought as much as possible into the waking consciousness. For in a Yoga which embraces all life completely and without reserve, the full use of Samadhi comes only when its gains can be made the normal possession and experience for an integral waking of the embodied soul in the human being.

---

1. *icchā-mṛtyu*.

# HATHAYOGA

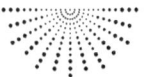

THERE are almost as many ways of arriving at Samadhi as there are different paths of Yoga. Indeed so great is the importance attached to it, not only as a supreme means of arriving at the highest consciousness, but as the very condition and status of that highest consciousness itself, in which alone it can be completely possessed and enjoyed while we are in the body, that certain disciplines of Yoga look as if they were only ways of arriving at Samadhi. All Yoga is in its nature an attempt and an arriving at unity with the Supreme,—unity with the being of the Supreme, unity with the consciousness of the Supreme, unity with the bliss of the Supreme,—or, if we repudiate the idea of absolute unity, at least at some kind of union, even if it be only for the soul to live in one status and periphery of being with the Divine, *sālokya,* or in a sort of indivisible proximity, *sāmīpya.* This can only be gained by rising to a higher level and intensity of consciousness than our ordinary mentality possesses. Samadhi, as we have seen, offers itself as the natural status of such a higher level and greater intensity. It assumes naturally a great importance in the Yoga of knowledge, because there it is the very principle of its method and its object to raise the mental consciousness into a clarity and concentrated power by which it can become entirely aware of, lost in, identified with true being. But there are two great disciplines in which it becomes of an even greater importance. To these two systems, to Rajayoga and Hathayoga, we may as well now turn; for in spite of the wide difference of their methods from that of the path of knowledge, they have this same principle as their final justification. At the same time, it will not be necessary for us to do more than regard the spirit of their gradations in passing; for in a synthetic and integral Yoga they take a secondary importance; their aims have indeed to be included, but their methods can either altogether be dispensed with or used only for a preliminary or else a casual assistance.

Hathayoga is a powerful, but difficult and onerous system whose whole principle of action is founded on an intimate connection between the body and the soul. The body is the key, the body the secret both of bondage and of release, of animal weakness and of divine power, of the obscuration of the mind and soul and of their illumination, of subjection to pain and limitation and of self-mastery, of death and of immortality. The body is not to the Hathayogin a mere mass of living matter, but a mystic bridge between the spiritual and the physical being; one has even seen an ingenious exegete of the Hathayogic discipline explain the Vedantic symbol OM as a figure of this mystic human body. Although, however, he speaks always of the physical body and makes that the basis of his practices, he does not view it with the eye of the anatomist or physiologist, but describes and explains it in language which always looks back to the subtle body behind the physical system. In fact the whole aim of the Hathayogin may be summarised from our point of view, though he would not himself put it in that language, as an attempt by fixed scientific processes to give to the soul in the physical body the power, the light, the purity, the freedom, the ascending scales of spiritual experience which would naturally be open to it, if it dwelt here in the subtle and the developed causal vehicle.

To speak of the processes of Hathayoga as scientific may seem strange to those who associate the idea of science only with the superficial phenomena of the physical universe apart from all that is behind them; but they are equally based on definite experience of laws and their workings and give, when rightly practised, their well-tested results. In fact, Hathayoga is, in its own way, a system of knowledge; but while the proper Yoga of knowledge is a philosophy of being put into spiritual practice, a psychological system, this is a science of being, a psycho-physical system. Both produce physical, psychic and spiritual results; but because they stand at different poles of the same truth, to one the psycho-physical results are of small importance, the pure psychic and spiritual alone matter, and even the pure psychic are only accessories of the spiritual which absorb all the attention; in the other the physical is of immense importance, the psychical a considerable fruit, the spiritual the highest and consummating result, but it seems for a long time a thing postponed and remote, so great and absorbing is the attention which the body demands. It must not be forgotten, however, that both do arrive at the same end. Hathayoga, also, is a path, though by a long, difficult and meticulous movement, *duḥkham āptum*, to the Supreme.

All Yoga proceeds in its method by three principles of practice; first, purification, that is to say, the removal of all aberrations, disorders, obstructions brought about by the mixed and irregular action of the energy of being in our physical, moral and mental system; secondly, concentration, that is to say, the bringing to its full intensity and the mastered and self-directed employment of that energy of being in us for a definite end; thirdly, liberation, that is to say, the release of our being from the narrow and painful knots of the individualised energy in a false and limited play, which at present are the law of our nature. The enjoyment of our liberated being which brings us into unity or union with the Supreme, is the consummation; it is that for which Yoga is done. Three indispensable steps and the high, open and infinite levels to which they mount; and in all its practice Hathayoga keeps these in view.

The two main members of its physical discipline, to which the others are mere accessories, are *āsana*, the habituating of the body to certain attitudes of immobility, and *prāṇāyāma*, the regulated direction and arrestation by exercises of breathing of the vital currents of energy in the body. The physical being is the instrument; but the physical being is made up of two elements, the physical and the vital, the body which is the apparent instrument and the basis, and the life energy, *prāṇa*, which is the power and the real instrument. Both of these instruments are now our masters. We are subject to the body, we are subject to the life energy; it is only in a very limited degree that we can, though souls, though mental beings, at all pose as their masters. We are bound by a poor and limited physical nature, we are bound consequently by a poor and limited life-power which is all that the body can bear or to which it can give scope. Moreover, the action of each and both in us is subject not only to the narrowest limitations, but to a constant impurity, which renews itself every time it is rectified, and to all sorts of disorders, some of which are normal, a violent order, part of our ordinary physical life, others abnormal, its maladies and disturbances. With all this Hathayoga has to deal; all this it has to overcome; and it does it mainly by these two methods, complex and cumbrous in action, but simple in principle and effective.

The Hathayogic system of Asana has at its basis two profound ideas which bring with them many effective implications. The first is that of control by physical immobility, the second is that of power by immobility. The power of physical immobility is as important in Hathayoga as the power of mental immobility in the Yoga of knowledge, and for parallel reasons. To the mind unaccustomed to the deeper truths of our being and nature they would both seem to be a seeking after the listless passivity of inertia. The direct contrary is the truth; for Yogic passivity, whether of mind or body, is a condition of the greatest increase, possession and continence of energy. The normal activity of our minds is for the most part a disordered restlessness, full of waste and rapidly tentative expenditure of energy in which only a little is selected for the workings of the self-mastering will,—waste, be it understood, from this point of view, not that of universal Nature in which what is to us waste, serves the purposes of her economy. The activity of our bodies is a similar restlessness.

It is the sign of a constant inability of the body to hold even the limited life energy that enters into or is generated in it, and consequently of a general dissipation of this Pranic force with a quite subordinate element of ordered and well-economised activity. Moreover in the consequent interchange and balancing between the movement and interaction of the vital energies normally at work in the body and their interchange with those which act upon it from outside, whether the energies of others or of the general Pranic force variously active in the environment, there is a constant precarious balancing and adjustment which may at any moment go wrong. Every obstruction, every defect, every excess, every lesion creates impurities and disorders. Nature manages it all well enough for her own purposes, when left to herself; but the moment the blundering mind and will of the human being interfere with her habits and her vital instincts and intuitions, especially when they create false or artificial habits, a still more precarious order and frequent derangement become the rule of the being. Yet this interference is inevitable, since man lives not for the purposes of the vital Nature in him alone, but for higher purposes which she had not contemplated in her first balance and to which she has with difficulty to adjust her operations. Therefore the first necessity of a greater status or action is to get rid of this disordered restlessness, to still the activity and to regulate it. The Hathayogin has to bring about an abnormal poise of status and action of the body and the life energy, abnormal not in the direction of greater disorder, but of superiority and self-mastery.

The first object of the immobility of the Asana is to get rid of the restlessness imposed on the body and to force it to hold the Pranic energy instead of dissipating and squandering it. The experience in the practice of Asana is not that of a cessation and diminution of energy by inertia, but of a great increase, inpouring, circulation of force. The body, accustomed to work off superfluous energy by movement, is at first ill able to bear this increase and this retained inner action and betrays it by violent tremblings; afterwards it habituates itself and, when the Asana is conquered, then it finds as much ease in the posture, however originally difficult or unusual to it, as in its easiest attitudes sedentary or recumbent. It becomes increasingly capable of holding whatever amount of increased vital energy is brought to bear upon it without needing to spill it out in movement, and this increase is so enormous as to seem illimitable, so that the body of the perfected Hathayogin is capable of feats of endurance, force, unfatigued expenditure of energy of which the normal physical powers of man at their highest would be incapable. For it is not only able to hold and retain this energy, but to bear its possession of the physical system and its more complete movement through it. The life energy, thus occupying and operating in a powerful, unified movement on the tranquil and passive body, freed from the restless balancing between the continent power and the contained, becomes a much greater and more effective force. In fact, it seems then rather to contain and possess and use the body than to be contained, possessed and used by it, —just as the restless active mind seems to seize on and use irregularly and imperfectly whatever spiritual force comes into it, but the tranquillised mind is held, possessed and used by the spiritual force.

The body, thus liberated from itself, purified from many of its disorders and irregularities, becomes, partly by Asana, completely by combined Asana and Pranayama, a perfected instrument. It is freed from its ready liability to fatigue; it acquires an immense power of health; its tendencies of decay, age and death are arrested. The Hathayogin even at an age advanced beyond the ordinary span maintains the unimpaired vigour, health and youth of the life in the body; even the appearance of physical youth is sustained for a longer time. He has a much greater power of longevity, and from his point of view, the body being the instrument, it is a matter of no small importance to preserve it long and to keep it for all that time free from impairing deficiencies. It is to be observed, also, that there are an enormous variety of Asanas in Hathayoga, running in their fullness beyond the number of eighty, some of them of the most complicated and difficult character. This variety serves partly to increase the results already noted, as well as to give a greater freedom and flexibility to the use of the body, but it serves also to alter the relation of the physical energy in the body to the earth energy with which it is related. The lightening of the heavy hold of the latter, of which the overcoming of fatigue is the first sign and the phenomenon of *utthāpana* or partial levitation the last, is one result. The gross body begins to acquire something of the nature of the subtle body and to possess something of its relations with the life-energy; that becomes a greater force more powerfully felt and yet capable of a lighter and freer and more resolvable physical action, powers which culminate in the Hathayogic *siddhis* or extraordinary powers of *garimā, mahimā, aṇimā* and *laghimā*.

Moreover, the life ceases to be entirely dependent on the action of the physical organs and functionings, such as the heart-beats and the breathing. These can in the end be suspended without cessation of or lesion to the life.

All this, however, the result in its perfection of Asana and Pranayama, is only a basic physical power and freedom. The higher use of Hathayoga depends more intimately on Pranayama. Asana deals more directly with the more material part of the physical totality, though here too it needs the aid of the other; Pranayama, starting from the physical immobility and self-holding which is secured by Asana, deals more directly with the subtler vital parts, the nervous system. This is done by various regulations of the breathing, starting from equality of respiration and inspiration and extending to the most diverse rhythmic regulations of both with an interval of inholding of the breath. In the end the keeping in of the breath, which has first to be done with some effort, and even its cessation become as easy and seem as natural as the constant taking in and throwing out which is its normal action. But the first objects of the Pranayama are to purify the nervous system, to circulate the life-energy through all the nerves without obstruction, disorder or irregularity, and to acquire a complete control of its functionings, so that the mind and will of the soul inhabiting the body may be no longer subject to the body or life or their combined limitations. The power of these exercises of breathing to bring about a purified and unobstructed state of the nervous system is a known and well-established fact of our physiology. It helps also to clear the physical system, but is not entirely effective at first on all its canals and openings; therefore the Hathayogin uses supplementary physical methods for clearing them out regularly of all their accumulations. The combination of these with Asana,—particular Asanas have even an effect in destroying particular diseases,—and with Pranayama maintains perfectly the health of the body. But the principal gain is that by this purification the vital energy can be directed anywhere, to any part of the body and in any way or with any rhythm of its movement.

The mere function of breathing into and out of the lungs is only the most sensible, outward and seizable movement of the Prana, the Breath of Life in our physical system. The Prana has according to Yogic science a fivefold movement pervading all the nervous system and the whole material body and determining all its functionings. The Hathayogin seizes on the outward movement of respiration as a sort of key which opens to him the control of all these five powers of the Prana. He becomes sensibly aware of their inner operations, mentally conscious of his whole physical life and action. He is able to direct the Prana through all the *nāḍīs* or nerve-channels of his system. He becomes aware of its action in the six *cakras* or ganglionic centres of the nervous system, and is able to open it up in each beyond its present limited, habitual and mechanical workings. He gets, in short, a perfect control of the life in the body in its most subtle nervous as well as in its grossest physical aspects, even over that in it which is at present involuntary and out of the reach of our observing consciousness and will. Thus a complete mastery of the body and the life and a free and effective use of them established upon a purification of their workings is founded as a basis for the higher aims of Hathayoga.

All this, however, is still a mere basis, the outward and inward physical conditions of the two instruments used by Hathayoga. There still remains the more important matter of the psychical and spiritual effects to which they can be turned. This depends on the connection between the body and the mind and spirit and between the gross and the subtle body on which the system of Hathayoga takes its stand. Here it comes into line with Rajayoga, and a point is reached at which a transition from the one to the other can be made.

# RAJAYOGA

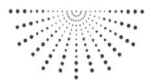

AS THE body and the Prana are the key of all the closed doors of the Yoga for the Hathayogin, so is the mind the key in Rajayoga. But since in both the dependence of the mind on the body and the Prana is admitted, in the Hathayoga totally, in the established system of Rajayoga partially, therefore in both systems the practice of Asana and Pranayama is included; but in the one they occupy the whole field, in the other each is limited only to one simple process and in their unison they are intended to serve only a limited and intermediate office. We can easily see how largely man, even though in his being an embodied soul, is in his earthly nature the physical and vital being and how, at first sight at least, his mental activities seem to depend almost entirely on his body and his nervous system. Modern Science and psychology have even held, for a time, this dependence to be in fact an identity; they have tried to establish that there is no such separate entity as mind or soul and that all mental operations are in reality physical functionings. Even otherwise, apart from this untenable hypothesis, the dependence is so exaggerated that it has been supposed to be an altogether binding condition, and any such thing as the control of the vital and bodily functionings by the mind or its power to detach itself from them has long been treated as an error, a morbid state of the mind or a hallucination. Therefore the dependence has remained absolute, and

Science neither finds nor seeks for the real key of the dependence and therefore can discover for us no secret of release and mastery.

The psycho-physical science of Yoga does not make this mistake. It seeks for the key, finds it and is able to effect the release; for it takes account of the psychical or mental body behind of which the physical is a sort of reproduction in gross form, and is able to discover thereby secrets of the physical body which do not appear to a purely physical enquiry. This mental or psychical body, which the soul keeps even after death, has also a subtle pranic force in it corresponding to its own subtle nature and substance,—for wherever there is life of any kind, there must be the pranic energy and a substance in which it can work,—and this force is directed through a system of numerous channels, called *nāḍī*,—the subtle nervous organisation of the psychic body,—which are gathered up into six (or really seven) centres called technically lotuses or circles, *cakra*, and which rise in an ascending scale to the summit where there is the thousand-petalled lotus from which all the mental and vital energy flows. Each of these lotuses is the centre and the storing-house of its own particular system of psychological powers, energies and operations,—each system corresponding to a plane of our psychological existence,—and these flow out and return in the stream of the pranic energies as they course through the *nād.īs*.

This arrangement of the psychic body is reproduced in the physical with the spinal column as a rod and the ganglionic centres as the chakras which rise up from the bottom of the column, where the lowest is attached, to the brain and find their summit in the *brahmarandhra* at the top of the skull. These chakras or lotuses, however, are in physical man closed or only partly open, with the consequence that only such powers and only so much of them are active in him as are sufficient for his ordinary physical life, and so much mind and soul only is at play as will accord with its need. This is the real reason, looked at from the mechanical point of view, why the embodied soul seems so dependent on the bodily and nervous life,—though the dependence is neither so complete nor so real as it seems. The whole energy of the soul is not at play in the physical body and life, the secret powers of mind are not awake in it, the bodily and nervous energies predominate. But all the while the supreme energy is there, asleep; it is said to be coiled up and slumbering like a snake,—therefore it is called the *kuḍḍalinī śakti*,—in the lowest of the chakras, in the *mūlādhāra*. When by Pranayama the division between the upper and lower prana currents in the body is dissolved, this Kundalini is struck and awakened, it uncoils itself and begins to rise upward like a fiery serpent breaking open each lotus as it ascends until the Shakti meets the Purusha in the *brahmarandhra* in a deep samadhi of union.

Put less symbolically, in more philosophical though perhaps less profound language, this means that the real energy of our being is lying asleep and inconscient in the depths of our vital system, and is awakened by the practice of Pranayama. In its expansion it opens up all the centres of our psychological being in which reside the powers and the consciousness of what would now be called perhaps our subliminal self; therefore as each centre of power and consciousness is opened up, we get access to successive psychological planes and are able to put ourselves in communication with the worlds or cosmic states of being which correspond to them; all the psychic powers abnormal to physical man, but natural to the soul develop in us. Finally, at the summit of the ascension, this arising and expanding energy meets with the superconscient self which sits concealed behind and above our physical and mental existence; this meeting leads to a profound samadhi of union in which our waking consciousness loses itself in the superconscient. Thus by the thorough and unremitting practice of Pranayama the Hathayogin attains in his own way the psychic and spiritual results which are pursued through more directly psychical and spiritual methods in other Yogas. The one mental aid which he conjoins with it, is the use of the mantra, sacred syllable, name or mystic formula which is of so much importance in the Indian systems of Yoga and common to them all. This secret of the power of the mantra, the six chakras and the Kundalini Shakti is one of the central truths of all that complex psycho-physical science and practice of which the Tantric philosophy claims to give us a rationale and the most complete compendium of methods. All religions and disciplines in India which use largely the psycho-physical method, depend more or less upon it for their practices.

Rajayoga also uses the Pranayama and for the same principal psychic purposes as the Hathayoga, but being in its whole principle a psychical system, it employs it only as one stage in the series of its practices and to a very limited extent, for three or four large utilities. It does not start with Asana and Pranayama, but insists first on a moral purification of the mentality. This preliminary is of supreme importance; without it the course of the rest of the Rajayoga is likely to be troubled, marred and full of unexpected mental, moral and physical perils.[1] This moral purification is divided in the established system under two heads, five *yamas* and five *niyamas*. The first are rules of moral self-control in conduct such as truth-speaking, abstinence from injury or killing, from theft etc.; but in reality these must be regarded as merely certain main indications of the general need of moral self-control and purity. *Yama* is, more largely, any self-discipline by which the rajasic egoism and its passions and desires in the human being are conquered and quieted into perfect cessation. The object is to create a moral calm, a void of the passions, and so prepare for the death of egoism in the rajasic human being. The *niyamas* are equally a discipline of the mind by regular practices of which the highest is meditation on the divine Being, and their object is to create a sattwic calm, purity and preparation for concentration upon which the secure pursuance of the rest of the Yoga can be founded.

It is here, when this foundation has been secured, that the practice of Asana and Pranayama come in and can then bear their perfect fruits. By itself the control of the mind and moral being only puts our normal consciousness into the right preliminary condition; it cannot bring about that evolution or manifestation of the higher psychic being which is necessary for the greater aims of Yoga. In order to bring about this manifestation the present nodus of the vital and physical body with the mental being has to be loosened and the way made clear for the ascent through the greater psychic being to the union with the superconscient Purusha. This can be done by Pranayama.

Asana is used by the Rajayoga only in its easiest and most natural position, that naturally taken by the body when seated and gathered together, but with the back and head strictly erect and in a straight line, so that there may be no deflection of the spinal cord. The object of the latter rule is obviously connected with the theory of the six chakras and the circulation of the vital energy between the *mūlādhāra* and the *brahmarandhra*. The Rajayogic Pranayama purifies and clears the nervous system; it enables us to circulate the vital energy equally through the body and direct it also where we will according to need, and thus maintain a perfect health and soundness of the body and the vital being; it gives us control of all the five habitual operations of the vital energy in the system and at the same time breaks down the habitual divisions by which only the ordinary mechanical processes of the vitality are possible to the normal life. It opens entirely the six centres of the psycho-physical system and brings into the waking consciousness the power of the awakened Shakti and the light of the unveiled Purusha on each of the ascending planes. Coupled with the use of the mantra it brings the divine energy into the body and prepares for and facilitates that concentration in Samadhi which is the crown of the Rajayogic method.

Rajayogic concentration is divided into four stages; it commences with the drawing both of the mind and senses from outward things, proceeds to the holding of the one object of concentration to the exclusion of all other ideas and mental activities, then to the prolonged absorption of the mind in this object, finally, to the complete ingoing of the consciousness by which it is lost to all outward mental activity in the oneness of Samadhi. The real object of this mental discipline is to draw away the mind from the outward and the mental world into union with the divine Being. Therefore in the first three stages use has to be made of some mental means or support by which the mind, accustomed to run about from object to object, shall fix on one alone, and that one must be something which represents the idea of the Divine. It is usually a name or a form or a mantra by which the thought can be fixed in the sole knowledge or adoration of the Lord. By this concentration on the idea the mind enters from the idea into its reality, into which it sinks silent, absorbed, unified. This is the traditional method. There are, however, others which are equally of a Rajayogic character, since they use the mental and psychical being as key. Some of them are directed rather to the quiescence of the mind than to its immediate absorption, as the discipline by which the mind is simply watched and allowed to exhaust its habit of vagrant thought in a purposeless running from which it feels all sanction, purpose and interest withdrawn, and that, more strenuous and rapidly effective, by which all outward-going thought is excluded and the mind forced to sink into itself where in its absolute quietude it can only reflect the pure Being or pass away into its superconscient existence. The method differs, the object and the result are the same.

Here, it might be supposed, the whole action and aim of Rajayoga must end. For its action is the stilling of the waves of consciousness, its manifold activities, *cittavṛtti*, first, through a habitual replacing of the turbid rajasic activities by the quiet and luminous sattwic, then, by the stilling of all activities; and its object is to enter into silent communion of soul and unity with the Divine. As a matter of fact we find that the system of Rajayoga includes other objects,—such as the practice and use of occult powers,—some of which seem to be unconnected with and even inconsistent with its main purpose. These powers or siddhis are indeed frequently condemned as dangers and distractions which draw away the Yogin from his sole legitimate aim of divine union. On the way, therefore, it would naturally seem as if they ought to be avoided; and once the goal is reached, it would seem that they are then frivolous and superfluous. But Rajayoga is a psychic science and it includes the attainment of all the higher states of consciousness and their powers by which the mental being rises towards the superconscient as well as its ultimate and supreme possibility of union with the Highest. Moreover, the Yogin, while in the body, is not always mentally inactive and sunk in Samadhi, and an account of the powers and states which are possible to him on the higher planes of his being is necessary to the completeness of the science.

These powers and experiences belong, first, to the vital and mental planes above this physical in which we live, and are natural to the soul in the subtle body; as the dependence on the physical body decreases, these abnormal activities become possible and even manifest themselves without being sought for. They can be acquired and fixed by processes which the science gives, and their use then becomes subject to the will; or they can be allowed to develop of themselves and used only when they come, or when the Divine within moves us to use them; or else, even though thus naturally developing and acting, they may be rejected in a single-minded devotion to the one supreme goal of the Yoga. Secondly, there are fuller, greater powers belonging to the supramental planes which are the very powers of the Divine in his spiritual and supramentally ideative being. These cannot be acquired at all securely or integrally by personal effort, but can only come from above, or else can become natural to the man if and when he ascends beyond mind and lives in the spiritual being, power, consciousness and ideation. They then become, not abnormal and laboriously acquired siddhis, but simply the very nature and method of his action, if he still continues to be active in the world-existence.

On the whole, for an integral Yoga the special methods of Rajayoga and Hathayoga may be useful at times in certain stages of the progress, but are not indispensable. It is true that their principal aims must be included in the integrality of the Yoga; but they can be brought about by other means. For the methods of the integral Yoga must be mainly spiritual, and dependence on physical methods or fixed psychic or psychophysical processes on a large scale would be the substitution of a lower for a higher action. We shall have occasion to touch upon this question later when we come to the final principle of synthesis in method to which our examination of the different Yogas is intended to lead.

---

1. In modern India people attracted to Yoga, but picking up its processes from books or from persons only slightly acquainted with the matter, often plunge straight into Pranayama of Rajayoga, frequently with disastrous results. Only the very strong in spirit can afford to make mistakes in this path.

ALSO BY SRI AUROBINDO

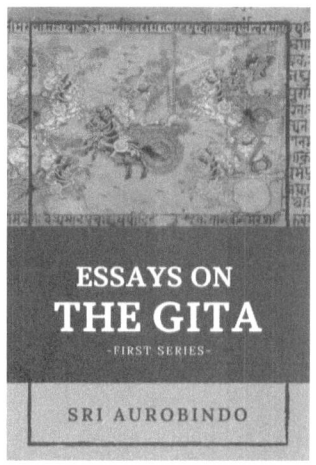

ESSAYS ON THE GITA

**FIRST SERIES**

- ISBN PAPERBACK: 9782357286313
- ISBN HARDCOVER: 9782357286320
- ISBN E-BOOK: 9782357286337

**SECOND SERIES**

- ISBN PAPERBACK: 9782357286481
- ISBN HARDCOVER: 9782357286498
- ISBN E-BOOK: 9782357286504

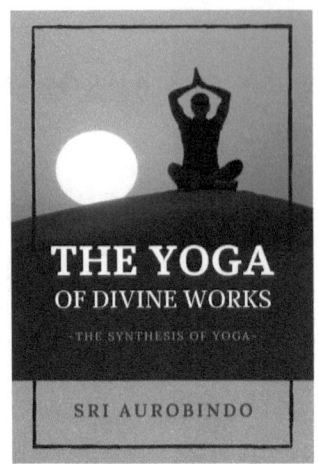

THE YOGA OF DIVINE WORKS

- ISBN PAPERBACK: 9782357286511
- ISBN HARDCOVER: 9782357286528
- ISBN E-BOOK: 9782357286535

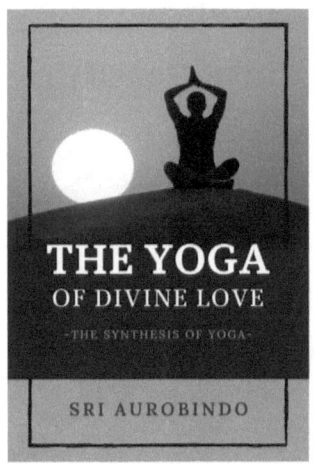

THE YOGA OF DIVINE LOVE

- ISBN PAPERBACK: 9782357286870
- ISBN HARDCOVER: 9782357286887
- ISBN E-BOOK: 9782357286894

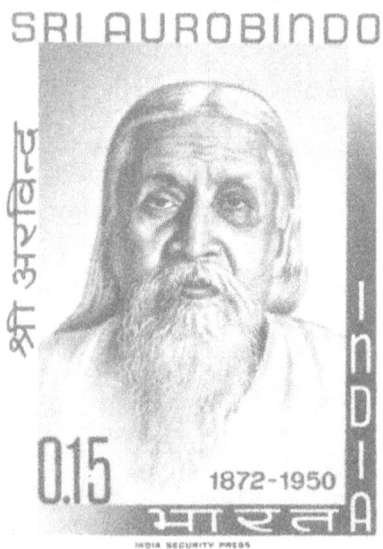

Copyright © 2021 by ALICIA EDITIONS
Credits: Canva
All rights reserved.
No part of this book may be reproduced in any form or by any electronic or mechanical means, including information storage and retrieval systems, without written permission from the author, except for the use of brief quotations in a book review.

www.ingramcontent.com/pod-product-compliance
Lightning Source LLC
LaVergne TN
LVHW040136080526
838202LV00042B/2926